Breast Massage after Implant and Explant Plastic Surgery

-The Study Guide-

Disclaimer and Terms of Use: No information contained in this book should be considered as medical advice. Your reliance upon information and content obtained by you at or through this publication is solely at your own risk. Solace Massage and Mindfulness or the author assumes no liability or responsibility for damage or injury to you, other persons, or property arising from any use of any product, information, idea, or instruction contained in the content or services provided to you through this book. Reliance upon information contained in this material is solely at the reader's own risk. The author has no financial interest in and receives no compensation from manufacturers of products or websites mentioned in this book.

ISBN-13: 978-1-7328066-9-6

ISBN: 1-7328066-9-1

Important Notes:

The information discussed in this book was compiled through reviewing research studies and published literature on breast surgery, interviewing experts, and listening to clients. Experts may disagree, and scientific advances may render some of this information outdated.

Table of Contents

Breast Massage Laws, Ordinances, and Standards of Practice

We will learn about breast massage as part of postoperative care after medical procedures, with a prescription or referral from a physician. Please ensure you meet state licensing board requirements for practicing breast massage in your state. Taking an online class (or reading a book) does not automatically mean you can perform breast massage in your state.

Many massage therapists are prohibited from touching "Specified Anatomical Areas," including the "area of the female breast that includes the areola and the nipple" (ORDINANCE NO. 10102 (N.S.), 2010). We will learn about manipulating the soft tissue structure of the upper torso, shoulders, and breast (not including the areola). Massage therapists can incorporate these techniques into a full-body or upper-body-focused massage session.

If you are Board Certified in Therapeutic Massage and Bodywork, according to Standard VI(h), you must "only provide therapeutic breast massage: (i) as indicated in the plan of care; (ii) after receiving informed, voluntary written consent; and (iii) only if the Certificant is permitted to do so under state law" (Standards of Practice, 2017).

In the State of California, for example, "providing massage of female breasts without the written consent of the person receiving the massage and a referral from a licensed California health care provider" is a violation of the Massage Therapy Act 2023 (Massage Therapy Act 2023, 2023).

Notes:

Why do clients get breast implant surgery?

Around 300,000 people have breast implant surgery each year in the United States. The article 'The Psychological Impact of Aesthetic Surgery: A Mini-Review' states that "there are a significant number of psychological factors that go into deciding whether to undergo this operation and then handling the recovery process. Prior to the operation, women may suffer from some degree of body image dissatisfaction that, if severe, can qualify as a psychological condition termed body dysmorphic disorder" (Jones et al., 2022).

People have a variety of reasons that motivate them to get breast implant-related surgery to change the appearance of their breasts. Individuals can also opt for a breast lift after aging, weight loss, pregnancy, and/or breastfeeding has changed the appearance of their breasts. Breast implant surgery may also be a part of gender affirmation surgery or breast cancer reconstruction. Breast implants do not last forever, and every year, many people choose to have their breast implants removed and replaced with new implants in the same size, a different size, or no implants at all.

Notes:

Why do clients benefit from massage after breast implant or explant surgery?

Many surgeons recommend self-massage after breast implant surgery, but clients are often hesitant or unsure of how to self-massage. Massage therapists can provide massage to reduce pain and swelling and show clients how to comfortably self-massage between visits. Back and neck massage delivered while the client is supine can also reduce stiff, sore muscles due to having a heavy breast implant and/or the client's post-surgery sleeping position. Clients may also have limited range of motion in their shoulder girdle after surgery. Clients may hesitate to receive regular massage from their usual massage therapist while healing. We can incorporate relaxation-focused massage techniques to help them with their aches and pains during the postoperative period.

Breast Anatomy Review

This class is about massage of the breast and upper torso. Let's briefly review the anatomy of the breast. Briot et al. state that the breast "originates in its upper part at the level of the clavicle and ends in its lower part at the level of the sixth rib. Laterally, the breast is located between the sternum and the lateral part of the rib cage starting from the axillary hollow." Breast tissue "rests on the pectoralis muscles, which are attached to the ribs." There are two layers of fascia in the breast. Deep fascia "is located between the pectoral muscles and the breast volume (gland + adipose tissue) and the superficial fascia located between the skin and the breast volume." Cooper's ligaments are "a three-dimensional mesh forming pockets of adipose tissue" which support the shape and contour of the breast (Briot et al., 2022).

Notes:

Sketch an image illustrating the boundaries of the breast.

Massage Can Reduce Anxiety Before and After Surgery

Why is massage useful before surgery? Research has found that:

- "Massage reduces pain by muscle relaxation and enkephalins release. The powerful stimulus of massage is conducted faster than pain along nerve pathways to the brain so massage can block pain conduction at the peripheral points (gaits of pain) and relieve pain" (Wang et al., 2022). Enkephalins are peptides that help control the experience of pain.
- "Massage can increase the circulation of soft tissue so irritant substances including lactic acid and inflammatory substances are removed from the tissue" (Wang et al., 2022).
- "Massage reduces pain sensation by inducing a sense of wellbeing" (Wang et al., 2022).

What is the research about massage and anxiety levels before surgery? Several presurgical massage studies have been conducted, including:

- "A randomized, controlled trial (RCT) ... concluded that a 20-min massage therapy before and after operation significantly reduced anxiety" before the placement of a vascular access device (Wang et al., 2022).
- A 20-minute massage "for cardiovascular patients before percutaneous coronary intervention (PCI) reduced anxiety level and emergency response. Moreover, blood pressure, pain score, and heart rate after the operation were lower in comparison to the control group" (Wang et al., 2022).
- In another study on patients receiving a variety of procedures, including cholecystectomy, hysterectomy,

mass excision, and orthopedic hardware removal, "patients had one session of 30 min of massage therapy and 30 min of music listening before the operation" and the results were that "postoperative anxiety scores were lower in intervention groups compared with the control group" and "the combination of music and massage more effective than using massage or music alone in reducing postoperative anxiety" (Wang et al., 2022).

When should the client and their care team start thinking about reducing anxiety before surgery?

Importantly, Wang et al. report that "assessment of patients about the level of preoperative anxiety 1–2 weeks prior to the surgical procedure was more effective in alleviating the anxiety compared to the preoperative visit on the night before surgery" and conclude that "earlier assessment of anxiety is recommended which provides us the opportunity of earlier intervention and referral of patients with a higher level of anxiety for a psychological consultation" (Wang et al., 2022).

Reducing a client's pain levels can also affect their anxiety levels. Kehlet & Dahl state that "pain treatment should also reduce anxiety and provide subjective comfort. Furthermore, effective analgesia might help to blunt autonomic and somatic reflex responses and thus restore organ functions and enable mobilisation and food intake, thereby helping to improve postoperative outcome" (Kehlet & Dahl, 2003). Indeed, a study showed that "massage therapy was associated with decreased pain and with lower anxiety in the postoperative period when compared to the control group" for patients undergoing heart surgery (Miozzo et al., 2016).

Let's learn more about the role of massage in reducing pain after surgery.

Massage Can Reduce Pain After Breast Surgery

Why offer massage after surgery? The good news is that massage can reduce pain levels in our clients after all kinds of operations. According to the Society for Oncology Massage, "massage therapists are recognized by the Joint Commission, the Veterans Administration, the Centers for Medicare and Medicaid for their value in providing a non-pharmaceutical option for pain" (Oncology Massage Therapy Guidelines, 2023).

- Research has shown that something as simple as foot massage has been found to be "effective in postoperative pain management" for people recovering from breast surgery (Ucuzal & Kanan, 2014).
- In a different study, researchers found that a 20-minute body massage given on postoperative days 1-3 after breast reconstruction "provided favorable effects in patients recovering from reconstructive surgery following mastectomy for breast cancer" (Dion et al., 2016).
- Another study on the effect of massage on postsurgical mastectomy recipients found a "significant reduction in pain, stress, and muscle tension, as well as an increase in relaxation" (Drackley et al., 2012).
- A further study on massage therapy given in postoperative days 1-3 after breast reconstruction found that "massage therapy provides temporary benefit for various postoperative symptoms" (Dilaveri et al., 2020).

Though we will focus on massage right after surgery in this class, it's important to know that massage is not just helpful in the first days and weeks after surgery. Let's briefly look at a study on massage several months after breast surgery. Myofascial massage focuses on "fascial holds, stretching, stroking, and varied pressure to tissue at modified depths" (Massingill et al., 2018). If you have had in-person training in myofascial massage, this may be a modality to consider using on your clients between 3-18 months after surgery (during the maturation phase of healing).

This study focused on women who had undergone breast cancer surgery (biopsy, lumpectomy, mastectomy, or reconstruction) between 3–18 months prior to the study and were experiencing persistent pain or lack of mobility in their breast, chest, or shoulder area. Participants received "two 30-minute massages per week for eight weeks (total of 16 massages). Intervention participants received myofascial massage specific to the breast, chest, and shoulder of the affected side." Massages "included a variety of techniques aimed at reducing pain, inflammation, and tissue sensitivity" (Massingill et al., 2018).

The massage protocol involved the following techniques:

- skin glide,
- j stroking,
- vertical stroking,
- strumming,
- fascial stretch,
- circular friction,
- deep fascial release,
- arm pull,
- side latissimus dorsi stretch, and
- twisting.

(Massingill et al., 2018)

Massingill et al. found that "there were substantial improvements in pain, mobility, and overall health among intervention participants, but little change among control participants," who received an equal number of massages that excluded the breast, chest, and shoulder area. The researchers shared that "intervention participants also expressed satisfaction with the aesthetic effects that myofascial release had on the scar tissue, stating, "my breast is in the right spot" and concluded that "physicians should refer women with persistent pain or mobility issues for massage treatments" (Massingill et al., 2018).

If you would like to learn more about the techniques listed in the massage protocol, I recommend taking an in-person myofascial massage class. Jeanne Massingill, the first author of the study I quoted, is an NCBTMB-approved provider and offers a live class titled, 'Post Breast Scar Tissue Release.' Find more information on her class at the NCBTMB website.

For Lymphedema Therapists: A Word on Massage for Clients with Lymphedema

Will deeper pressure massage techniques affect clients who have lymphedema? It's important to note that a separate study of women with breast cancer-related lymphedema found that "excess lymphoedema volume decreased after three weeks of intensive treatment in both a group given MLD and a 'placebo MLD group' given "deep massage" including "relaxing transverse movements on the muscles of the ipsilateral neck, back, shoulder, arm and hand." Treatment consisted of "14 sessions of physiotherapy during the 3-week intensive phase" in addition to "education, skin care, compression therapy and exercises." The deeper massage techniques used in this study did not result in an increase in lymphedema volume - in fact, fluid volume decreased at rates equal to those given MLD (de Vrieze et al., 2022). I encourage massage therapists trained in caring for clients with lymphedema to look into classes offering training in fibrosis techniques for lymphedema.

Bottom line:

- People have a variety of reasons for getting breast implant-related surgery,
- Massage can affect anxiety levels before surgery,
- Massage can affect pain, mobility, and overall health after surgery, and
- Self-massage after breast implant surgery is recommended by many surgeons.

Now that we've considered the pain-relieving benefits of massage after surgery, let's look specifically at massage for clients after breast implant-related surgeries.

Notes:

What would you say to a regular massage client that asks if they could see you for massage before their breast implant related surgery?

Which study on massage before surgery is most interesting to you? Why?

Notes:

What is Breast Implant Surgery?

What are breast implants? According to the U.S. Food and Drug Administration (FDA), "breast implants are medical devices implanted under the breast tissue or chest muscle to increase breast size (augmentation) or to replace breast tissue that has been removed due to cancer or trauma, or that has failed to develop properly due to a severe breast abnormality (reconstruction). They are also used in revision surgeries, which seek to correct or improve the result of an original surgery."

What types of implants are used? The FDA states that "there are two types of breast implants approved for sale in the United States: saline-filled and silicone gel-filled. Both types have a silicone outer shell. They vary in size, shell thickness, shell surface texture, and shape (contour)." (Breast Implants, 2023).

Where are the incisions made for the breast implant surgery?

Incisions can be:

- Inframammary – in the crease underneath the breast,
- Periareolar - at the outer edge of the areola,
- Transabdominal – on the abdomen or
- Transaxillary – in the armpit.

Notes:

Using the image provided, label the different incisions used for breast implant surgery.

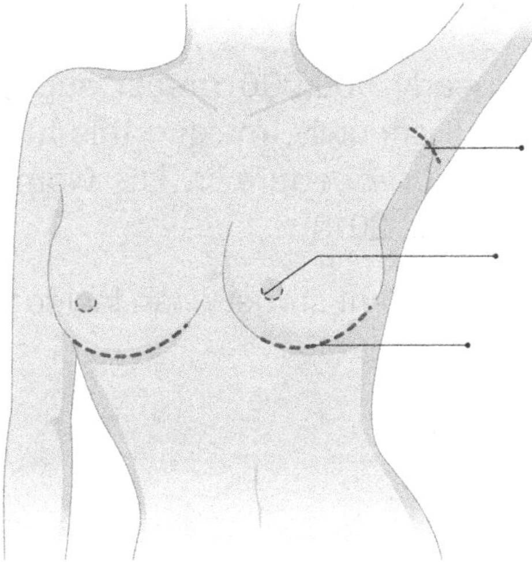

It's important to realize that not all breast implants are the same and not everyone has the newest model of breast implant. Our clients may have had implant surgery recently, or they may have implants that are decades old. Clients with older implants may not know the brand or shape or even if they are saline or silicone. Many clients with older implants believe that they are meant to last a lifetime.

It is estimated that "nearly 300,000 breast augmentation surgeries are performed annually, making this the second most common aesthetic procedure in US women (after liposuction)" (Coombs et al., 2019).

Complications of breast implant surgery can include:

- breast asymmetry,
- breastfeeding difficulty,
- breast implant illness,
- calcium deposits,
- capsular contracture,
- changes in nipple and breast sensation, including breast pain,
- extrusion,
- hematoma,
- infection,
- lymphadenopathy,,
- migration of implants,
- necrosis,
- palpability,
- rupture,
- seroma,

- scarring,
- tissue atrophy,
- visibility,
- delayed wound healing, and
- wrinkling/rippling.

We will look at some of these complications in more depth later in class.

What happens in breast implant surgery?

An article from the Cleveland Clinic states that "traditionally, plastic surgeons place breast implants either beneath the pectoralis major muscle (submuscular placement) or over the pectoralis but beneath the glandular breast parenchyma (subglandular placement)" (Coombs et al., 2019). The dual plane is a third placement for breast implants.

The advantages of submuscular placement are:

- "Smoother transition of the upper breast pole from the chest wall" (Coombs et al., 2019).
- "Less rippling visible through the skin, due to the additional muscular coverage of the implant" (Coombs et al., 2019).
- "Capsular contraction rates are lower with submuscular placement, likely due to possible contamination of implants by lactiferous ductal microbes when accessing the subglandular plane" (Coombs et al., 2019).

Disadvantages of submuscular placement include:

- "Pronounced discomfort after surgery" (Coombs et al., 2019).

- "Animation deformities with muscle contraction, particularly in young, highly active patients" (Coombs et al., 2019).
- "Athletes with submuscular implants seem to need longer periods to recover in comparison to those with subglandular implants" (Stamouli et al., 2023).

The pectoralis major (PM) muscle is affected during submuscular placement. Animation deformity was just mentioned, which is described as "implant displacement with pectoralis muscle contraction" (Fracol et al., 2019). How does this happen? Stamouli et al. state that "traditionally fixed volume implants and tissue expanders are placed at least partially under the PM so that a robust layer of tissue lies between the artificial material and the skin." The pectoralis major muscle is cut during surgery. Stamouli et al. state that "this procedure often involves the partial or even the complete division of the lower and the medial insertions of PM. The implant is then either partially covered by the muscle leaving the lower pole lying totally subcutaneously or simply covered by an ADM" (Stamouli et al., 2023). We will learn about Acellular Dermal Matrix (ADM) later in class.

What is the result of cutting the PM? Stamouli et al. state that the primary functions of the pectoralis major are "the flexion, adduction, and internal rotation of the humerus. The severance of its insertions - usually by trauma - compromises arm movements" (Stamouli et al., 2023).

What types of issues are caused? Stamouli et al. state that "imaging, including ultrasound shear wave elastography and volumetric MRI, showed that subpectoral implantation reduces the actual volume of the muscle and this effect persists for a long period of time; and that the clavicular region of PM contributes more to joint stiffness at rest and at flexion torques, indicating a need for compensation for the loss of the lower region of the PM" (Stamouli et al., 2023).

Stamouli et al. reviewed a study where isometric dynamometry of patients with a breast cancer history "who underwent 2-stage subpectoral reconstruction with disinsertion of sternocostal fibers ... showed that the subpectoral implant group was weaker in shoulder adduction and demonstrated lower shoulder stiffness during submaximal adduction torques" (Stamouli et al., 2023).

Coombs et al. note that "a popular modification of submuscular placement involves creating a surgical dissection plane between the subglandular tissue and the pectoralis major fascia. This "dual-plane" approach allows the parenchyma to retract superiorly and reduce breast ptosis." (Coombs et al., 2019). Ptosis is a medical term that refers to drooping or sagging. Parenchyma is a word for the tissue of an organ.

The PM is also affected in a dual plane breast implant surgery. Stamouli et al. reviewed a study where the isometric dynamometry of "20 women with bilateral breast augmentation with dual plane technique... showed reduced strength during adduction between baseline and 12 months and between 3 and 12 months for the operated individuals. Furthermore, a significant difference in muscle strength during adduction was noted among the groups at 12 months (Stamouli et al., 2023).

Notes:

Sketch the different types of breast implant placements, showing the differences between breast implants beneath the pectoralis major muscle (submuscular placement), breast implants over the pectoralis but beneath the glandular breast parenchyma (subglandular placement) and the dual plane approach.

Hauch et al. states that the "window shade deformity" happens with contraction of the inferior border of the pectoralis major muscle" and that performing a "limited capsulectomy over the anterior surface of the pectoralis major muscle" creates "soft tissue coverage at the lower pole of the breast and prevents window shading of the pectoralis major muscle" (Hauch et al., 2021).

Notes:

How would you describe 'dancing breast' and 'window shade' animation deformities to a client?

Notes:

What issues have you seen involving implant placement? What worked to correct these issues?

Notes:

Sketch the different types of ptosis.

What is the difference between severe ptosis and lower breast sagging?

Rippling

Rippling happens when folds of the breast implant become visible through the skin. Vidya et al. found that if reconstruction after breast cancer treatment involves prepectoral implant-based breast reconstruction using mesh "over time, and under the weight of the implant, the upper part of the prepectoral reconstruction atrophies. This, coupled with thinning of the collagen in the skin, can result in visible implant rippling. Indeed, subcutaneous cover influences the degree of rippling and is often less prevalent in those with a high body mass index (BMI)" (Vidya et al., 2019).

Notes:

Sketch an image of rippling.

Bottom line:

- Breast implants are medical devices.
- Breast implants have a silicone outer shell and can be filled with saline or silicone.
- Incisions can be inframammary, periareolar, transabdominal, or transaxillary.
- Breast implants can be placed under or over the pectoralis muscle or in a dual plane approach.
- The risk of rippling and capsular contracture may be lower when implants are placed under the pectoralis muscle.
- The risk of discomfort and animation deformity may be higher when implants are placed under the pectoralis muscle.
- Around 300,000 breast augmentation surgeries are performed annually.
- Prior to the operation, women may suffer from some degree of body image dissatisfaction that, if severe, can qualify as a psychological condition termed body dysmorphic disorder.
- Animation deformities can include dancing breast and window shade deformities.
- Complications of breast implant surgery include breast asymmetry, breastfeeding difficulty, breast implant illness, calcium deposits, capsular contracture, changes in nipple and breast sensation including breast pain, extrusion, hematoma, infection, lymphadenopathy, migration of implants, necrosis, palpability, rupture, seroma, scarring, tissue atrophy, visibility, delayed wound healing, and wrinkling.

Notes:

Breast Augmentation - Cosmetic

Why do people get breast implant surgery for cosmetic reasons? Swezey et al. state that "breast augmentation is a surgical procedure designed to enhance the size of the patient's breasts, using implants (saline or silicone) or fat transfer." Goals include increasing the size and projection of the breast. The researchers estimate that "approximately 3.5 million people in the United States have breast implants, making it one of the most commonly performed cosmetic surgical procedures" (Swezey et al., 2023).

Complications

After surgery, the patient may develop a hematoma, which is a "collection of blood near the surgical site. May cause swelling, bruising and pain. Hematomas usually occur soon after surgery but can occur any time there is injury to the breast. The body may absorb small hematomas, but large ones may require medical intervention, such as surgical draining." A seroma may also form, which is a "collection of fluid around the implant. May cause swelling, pain and bruising. The body may absorb small seromas. Large ones will require a surgical drain" (Risks and complications of breast implants, 2023). We will learn about medications that may increase the incidence of hematoma in the medications section of class.

Calcium deposits can also form, which feel like "hard lumps under the skin around the implant. These can be mistaken for cancer during mammography, resulting in additional surgery" (Risks and complications of breast implants, 2023).

Notes:

How would you explain to a client the difference between a hematoma and a seroma?

Notes:

What complications have you seen after breast augmentation? What helped to resolve them?

Breast Implant Replacement - Cosmetic

Clients may want to have their breast implants removed and replaced for a variety of reasons. They may want a different size of implant, or they may have experienced a complication with their previous implant or implants.

What are the top complications that may result in breast implants being removed and replaced with new implants?

After every breast implant surgery, the body forms a capsule around the breast implant. This fibrous capsule of scar tissue is "a normal reaction to the foreign implant" (Swezey et al., 2023). Unfortunately, "over a typical 15-y period, ~50% women who undergo breast augmentation or reconstruction surgery will experience complications or implant failure, including asymmetric appearance of the implant, pain, and capsular contracture (CC), with ~10% of these complications occurring within two to 4 y following surgery" (Guimier et al., 2022).

Capsular Contracture

Let's learn more about capsular contracture (CC). According to Guimier et al., "CC is defined as the formation of scar tissue—known as a fibrous capsule—around the breast implant during a heightened inflammatory response following surgery and is the second most common reason for follow-on operations." It's important to note that "while inflammatory responses are common with all implanted devices, the term 'capsular contracture' is reserved to describe contracture phenomena associated with breast implants" (Guimier et al., 2022).

How common is capsular contracture? A study of over 12,000 breast implants found that "the most common reason for breast implant revision in both groups was capsular contracture (4775 cosmetic revisions [37.1%]" (Lieffering et al., 2022).

What is happening in the body? We know that the body forms a capsule around the breast implant after surgery. "The foreign body response (FBR) is described as the host's response to implanted biomaterials, which involves a complex cascade of immune modulators." Sheng et al. explain that "macrophages, the main immune cells in FBR, infiltrated into the expanded tissue and located at the tissue-material interface from day 1-90. Following the decrease of the number of macrophages, collagen deposited, and fibroblasts transformed into myofibroblasts at the tissue-material interface, leading to the formation of a fibrous capsule from day 14" (Sheng et al., 2014).

What is the timeline of development of the normal capsule? Sheng et al. share that "fibrous tissue began to form around the tissue expander at day 14, increased to maximum at 30 days and decreased gradually with a persistent thin layer at day 90" (Sheng et al., 2014).

What goes wrong to form a capsular contracture? Susini et al. state that "when a breast implant is set, the immune system reacts physiologically by forming a thin fibrous capsule, which stabilizes the implant in place. The capsule normally does not exceed 1–1.5 mm, but in some cases, it undergoes a pathological fibrotic thickening process, leading to capsular contracture (CC). CC develops from a few months to several years after implant surgery" (Susini et al., 2023). The pressure of an implant on the body becomes more focused when capsular contracture occurs. Kim et al. state that chest wall depression can occur in patients with capsular contracture because the capsule can "induce the effect of constant pressure to one point by holding the implant in one place" (Kim et al., 2022).

How often does this happen? A study by de Bakker et al. states that "prevalence estimates for capsular contracture (CC) range from 5% to 19% for breast augmentation and 19% to 25% for breast reconstruction, although numbers vary between studies. Known risk factors include breast reconstructive surgery after breast cancer, irradiation of the breast, subglandular implant placement, postoperative hematoma" (de Bakker et al., 2023).

Capsular Contracture and Mast Cells

Mast cells may be a part of capsular contracture. Brazin et al. found that "symptomatic capsular contracture occurs in about 10 % of primary breast augmentations and in more than double that rate in reconstruction after mastectomy, especially in the setting of radiation. Mast cells, traditionally associated with immune response and inflammation, secrete profibrotic mediators and may play a role in capsule formation and contracture." The researchers collected capsule tissue "from patients who underwent exchange of tissue expanders for permanent implants, revision of reconstruction, or revision augmentation" and found that "within breast capsule tissue mast cells contain mediators that may activate neighboring fibroblasts" (Brazin et al., 2014). We will learn more about mast cells later in class.

A study found a link between capsular contracture and silicone particles. de Bakker et al. state that "common complications are still related to the capsule surrounding the implant. Capsule formation is a normal foreign body response, although excessive thickening and contracture are adverse reactions and may result in complaints experienced by the patient." They examined twenty-two capsules from 11 patients who only had complaints about one of their implants but had both removed and found that a "significant correlation between capsule silicone content and capsular contracture is shown. An extensive and continued foreign body response to silicone particles is likely to be responsible" (de Bakker et al., 2023). The researchers also mentioned a previous study that found that "Baker grade IV capsules, compared with Baker grade I capsules, were significantly thicker. They also expressed more CD68+ cells, indicating an increased influx of innate immune cells (eg, macrophages), which are characteristic of foreign-body granulomatous reactions observed in reaction to fillers" (de Bakker et al., 2023).

Capsular Contracture, Implant Placement and Biofilm

The location of implant placement and the type of implant used may also have an effect on the risk of capsular contracture. Coombs et al. state that "a meta-analysis from 17,000 implants found that the risk of capsular contracture was significantly higher when an implant was placed in a subglandular pocket than in a submuscular pocket and that although texturing decreased capsular contracture compared with smooth implants, the effect was modest when a textured or smooth implant was placed in a submuscular location. With regard to incision location, studies have reported that the incidence of capsular contracture is highest with transaxillary and periareolar incisions, and lowest with inframammary incisions. The leading theory is that contamination of the implant (primarily from the mammary ducts) results in biofilm formation" (Coombs et al., 2019). Breast implants can also be placed in the body during a tummy tuck. Stümpfle et al. performed a chart review of 68 patients who underwent breast augmentation through an abdominoplasty incision and found that a "transabdominal approach may decrease the risk of implant contamination because there is no contact of the implants with skin" (Stümpfle et al., 2021).

How does biofilm affect the breast implant capsule? Portillo et al. share that "the presence of bacteria growing as biofilm on the surface ... may cause persistent low-grade inflammation of the surrounding tissue, leading to formation of capsular fibrosis and subsequent contracture. A significant correlation between the degree of capsular contracture and the presence of biofilm on breast implants was demonstrated by several authors, especially when using a sonication technique." The researchers tested 112 breast implants and found that "fifty two of them had a positive sonication fluid culture (46%). Among positive sonication fluid cultures, *P. acnes* was isolated in most cases (54%). *P. acnes* seems to have a role, especially in Baker grade IV. Its origin is most likely the patient skin or colonized mammary ducts at the incision site" (Portillo et al., 2013). Flores et al. found that "most bacteria originated from the skin and were described as causative for capsule fibrosis" and specifically "in patients with aesthetic dissatisfaction, *S. epidermidis* was identified most frequently (75%)" (Flores et al., 2024). We will learn more about biofilm later in class.

Capsular contracture may be different in mastectomy reconstruction clients. Mohan et al. state that "Hirsch et al. recommended a nuanced change for irradiated patients to direct clinical management, adding an "R" to Baker grade to indicate involvement of deeper layers such as muscle or capsule, and "RS" to also indicate skin involvement. Moreover, in prepectoral reconstruction where an ADM is used and an actual capsule does not even form, any contracture that occurs following radiation therapy may be attributed to radiation-induced fibrosis of the skin, subcutaneous fat, ADM, or muscle rather than capsule" (Mohan et al., 2024).

Capsular Contracture Treatments

If clients have capsular contracture after their first set of implants, the surgeon may use an acellular dermal matrix (ADM) when placing a subsequent breast implant. We will learn more about this in the Breast Reconstruction after Cancer section.

Some clients opt to have liposuction and graft the harvested fat to the breast as an alternative treatment for capsular contracture (CC). Susini et al. state that "the surgeon can place a fat graft in the initial procedure and use lipofilling as an alternative CC treatment. Data showed that lipofilling was effective in ameliorating pain from capsular formation, as it reduced the foreign body sensation, the feeling of tension, and the feeling of cold breast. Haran et al. showed that fat grafting elevated the CC resolution rate of secondary procedures up to 86%" (Susini et al., 2023).

How else can fat grafting be used to improve the appearance of the breast? Davis et al. state that "fat grafting in aesthetic breast surgery may be performed as a form of primary autologous breast augmentation or as an adjunct to implant-based breast augmentation to disguise implant edges" (Davis et al., 2020).

Liposuction and fat grafting to the breast after breast implant surgery may help by:

- Reducing pain from capsular formation,
- Reducing feeling of tension,
- Reducing the feeling of cold breasts and
- Disguising implant edges.

Notes:

What is capsular contracture? What has your experience been with capsular contracture?

Implant Rupture

Sometimes, the implant can rupture. According to Swezey et al., "the extravasation of silicone outside of the fibrous capsule is called an extracapsular rupture." What may the client experience? Swezey et al. state that "in silicone prostheses, some degree of chest wall pain may be present as the granulomatous inflammatory reaction takes place." Specifically, "extracapsular silicone implant ruptures can sometimes produce a palpable mass or irregularity of the breast as inflammation and granulomatous tissue form; alternately, they may present with vague pain or tenderness symptoms or may be completely asymptomatic" (Swezey et al., 2023).

The rupture of older implants can cause scar tissue to form. Azis et al. state that "in an extracapsular rupture, silicone gel extravasates into the adjacent tissues, frequently in an infiltrative pattern that can result in a significant local tissue reaction and scar formation." It's valuable to ask the client when they had their breast implant surgery, as newer models of implants are made of cohesive silicone. Azis et al. state that "there is a difference between older silicone and newer, more cohesive silicone implants. Without certain exceptional circumstances, cohesive silicone will not spread to adjacent tissue; however, silicone present in older generations of implants is susceptible to widespread dissemination" (Azis et al., 2023).

What about saline? In saline implants, the rupture will result in a very noticeable loss in breast volume. Swezey et al. state that "in saline prostheses, apart from the diminution in breast volume, few other symptoms can be identified" (Swezey et al., 2023).

Swezey et al. have found that "the incidence of implant rupture increases with the age of the implant" and "breast implants are not permanent and have a definitive lifespan that varies from 12-35 years" (Swezey et al., 2023).

Flores et al. analyzed a total of 100 breast implant revisions in 66 patients and found a "correlation between implant complications and gram-positive bacteria found on breast implant surfaces. The most common implant-based complication seen at simultaneously positive samples was implant rupture in 50% of the authors' cases" (Flores et al., 2024). The authors conclude that "gram-positive bacteria might noticeably be involved in implant shell disruption through accelerated immunologic triggering. Thus, immunologic reactions may be more severe and perhaps accelerated in the case of bacterial contamination, which could increase the probability of implant shell degradation" (Flores et al., 2024).

What are physicians looking for in a suspected case of implant rupture? Swezey et al. state that "pertinent physical examination findings include:

- Breast shape and symmetry
- New breast masses
- Associated lymphadenopathy in the axillae or elsewhere
- The texture of the breast implant in question versus the contralateral breast implant
- Skin changes in the affected breast versus the contralateral breast
- Nipple discharge" (Swezey et al., 2023).

If a rupture is suspected, clients may have had ultrasound imaging of their implant and may mention the term 'snowstorm sign.' Swezey et al. state that "the snowstorm sign is a sonographic finding of silicone gel droplets mixed with breast tissue showing a heterogeneous echogenic appearance resulting from the dispersion of the ultrasound beam" (Swezey et al., 2023).

Notes:

What has your experience been with implant rupture?

Bottoming Out/Double Bubble

Two complications that involve breast implants that do require surgery but not new implants are called bottoming out and double bubble.

According to Wagner et al., bottoming out describes "the redistribution of breast volume from the upper pole to the lower pole of the breast" (Wagner et al., 2022).

Bresnick states that "double-bubble deformity is one of the most common problems in breast augmentation, with or without mastopexy" and that it occurs when "a breast implant sits lower than the old inframammary crease" (Bresnick, 2016).

Notes:

Sketch an image that shows the differences between double bubble and bottoming out.

Moving Breast Implant Placement From Subglandular to Submuscular

Hauch et al. state that "over the past 2 decades, we have seen an increasing number of long-term complications associated with subglandular breast augmentation in our practice and as reported by many plastic surgeons in various communities including Southern California. These include:

- inferior migration of the implant
- implant wrinkling
- capsular contracture
- enlarged areolas
- breast asymmetry" (Hauch et al., 2021).

The surgeons state that "subglandular to subpectoral site change represents an important tool for dealing with these implant-related complications. This concept, introduced in the mid-1990s by Maxwell, has evolved to include total or partial capsulectomy and, more recently, the use of acellular dermal matrix (ADM) or mesh" (Hauch et al., 2021).

Slide Down Deformity and Waterfall Deformity

Hauch et al. also describe "slide-down deformity" as a "unitary descent of the implant, breast tissue, and inframammary fold (IMF)" and state that "as part of a comprehensive approach to treating slide-down deformity, a mastopexy is performed concurrently" with subglandular to subpectoral site change of the breast implant (Hauch et al., 2021).

Sometimes also called "Snoopy breast," White & Peterson describe waterfall deformity as occurring "when breast tissue slides off a fixed structure or object or a combination of both. Conceptually, the waterfall deformity is when ptotic breast parenchyma falls off a breast implant and gives a striking and unnatural shape. This is seen in both cosmetic and reconstructive patients." Surgeons try to correct this by using "large implants to stretch the breast tissue so that it is thinner and tighter so that there is less "loose" tissue to hang off the implant. Another older and conservative approach to augmentation/mastopexy is to perform a delayed 2-stage procedure where the hanging tissue can be excised at the time of mastopexy" (White & Peterson, 2021).

What's the difference between these two complications? Hauch et al. explain that "Since IMF descent is not a hallmark of waterfall deformity or pseudoptosis, the key measurement defining slide-down deformity is, therefore, the SN-to-IMF distance, which will be longer than normal" (Hauch et al., 2021). SN is the sternal notch.

Notes:

Sketch an image that shows the differences between slide-down deformity and waterfall deformity.

Breast Implant Surgery After Massive Weight Loss

Weight loss can affect the breast shape as well as skin quality. Wagner et al. state that "changes in weight, and specifically weight loss, can contribute to secondary ptosis. With weight loss, there is a decrease in volume and deflation of the breasts" (Wagner et al., 2022).

According to Ramanadham et al., clients with breast implants after massive weight loss may have "poor skin elasticity and lack of a discrete IMF," and "recurrent ptosis and poor scarring remain common procedural outcomes." In one study, "implant malposition was observed in 61.9% of patients." Surgeons may use "an inverted-T resection, stabilization of the IMF with suturing to the periosteum, use of textured implants or implants with tabs for fixation, or use of acellular dermis" (Ramanadham et al., 2020).

Knowing that these clients are at risk for implant malposition and that the surgeon may have sutured the inframammary fold (IMF) to the periosteum, I would focus on manual lymphatic drainage to reduce swelling during the massage and minimize movement of the implant and inframammary fold. Hauch et al. states that "the IMF itself is a coalescence of thickened tissue from the skin and subcutaneous tissues to the periosteum" (Hauch et al., 2021). We do not want to loosen the stabilization with deeper massage techniques.

Notes:

What has your experience been with breast surgery after massive weight loss?

Breast Lift with Breast Implant

Patients may also have breast implants removed and replaced as part of a breast lift operation.

What is a breast lift, also known as mastopexy? According to Mowlavi et al., "the goals of mastopexy are to reshape the breast, redistribute volume, and reposition the nipple-areola complex" (Wagner et al., 2022). Researchers state that "a breast lift is indicated to accommodate the forecasted redundancy in skin and breast ptosis created by implant explantation. The most popular approaches to mastopexy include the inferior and superior pedicled breast lifts" (Mowlavi et al., 2023).

Ptosis is a medical term that refers to drooping or sagging, and according to Ramanadham et al., "can be classified using the Regnault classification system. This commonly used system describes ptosis by the relative position of the nipple–areolar complex (NAC) and the inframammary fold" The lower the nipple is below the inframammary fold, the more severe the grade of ptosis. (Ramanadham et al., 2020). The term pseudoptosis is used when the nipple is above the IMC, but the breast is still ptotic. Wagner et al. share that "ptosis and pseudoptosis of the breast can develop with normal aging, pregnancy, significant weight loss, and macromastia (Wagner et al., 2022). Macromastia is a term for abnormally large breasts.

Why do clients choose a particular type of breast surgery? Ramanadham et al. state that "if a patient is happy with the volume and upper pole fullness, a mastopexy alone may suffice. It is important to counsel the patient that a decrease of 1 cup size is expected with a mastopexy alone. However, if a patient instead desires restoration of upper pole volume or an increase in breast size, a mastopexy should be combined with an augmentation in a 1- or 2-stage manner, depending on the amount of nipple elevation and vertical excess" (Ramanadham et al., 2020).

According to Ramanadham et al., augmentation and mastopexy "is a good option for patients that lack volume and desire increased upper pole fullness or increased overall breast size. The addition of an implant is challenging because it creates 2 opposing forces. Augmentation increases volume and the skin envelope, while mastopexy repositions the nipple and removes excess skin. Together, tension on the wound increases, as well as gravitational forces on the breast. This can significantly compromise the NAC, especially with greater nipple movement and larger implants" (Ramanadham et al., 2020).

Notes:

Sketch and image that shows the difference between ptosis and pseudoptosis.

What Complications Are Seen in Each of the Different Types of Mastopexy?

Ramanadham et al. state that “the most common complications described are associated with circumareolar and inverted-T mastopexy techniques. In circumareolar mastopexies, areolar herniation, purse-string breakage, knot exposure, and a palpable ring are commonly observed... Other complications include widened scars and NAC, central flattening, and pleating ... Circumareolar mastopexies result in an overall complication rate of 41.5% compared with 9.7% in vertical mastopexies and 14% with an inverted-T resection. Circumareolar techniques also tend to have higher revision rates, while vertical have increased asymmetries, and inverted-T are seen to more commonly bottom out” (Ramanadham et al., 2020).

If a client has an inverted-T incision, I would be careful not to be too aggressive in pushing the breast tissue inferiorly to reduce the risk of my contributing to the implant bottoming out.

Bottom Line:

- Around 3.5 million people in the United States have breast implants.
- Over a typical 15-year period, □50% of women who undergo breast augmentation or reconstruction surgery will experience complications.
- Hematoma and seroma may need draining by the surgeon’s office.
- Calcification feels like hard lumps under the skin.
- A top reason for breast implant revision surgery is capsular contracture.

- Capsular contracture results from pathological fibrotic thickening.
- Mast cells, biofilm, and capsule silicone content may have a role in capsular contracture.
- Capsular contracture rates are highest with transaxillary and periareolar incisions and lowest with inframammary incisions.
- Risk factors for capsular contracture include irradiation of the breast, subglandular implant placement, and postoperative hematoma.
- Capsular contracture can be evaluated using the Baker Classification.
- Baker grade IV capsules are significantly thicker than Baker grade I capsules.
- Chest wall depression can occur in patients with capsular contracture due to constant pressure on one point.
- The risk of implant rupture increases with the age of the implant.
- Snowstorm sign is a sonographic finding of silicone gel droplets mixed with breast tissue.
- A stepladder sign is a sonographic finding of an intracapsular rupture of a silicone implant.
- Implant malposition may occur in over 60 percent of patients who have breast implants after massive weight loss.
- A double bubble happens when the breast implant sits lower than the old inframammary crease.
- Bottoming out refers to when breast volume is redistributed from the upper pole to the lower pole of the breast.

- The slide-down deformity is the unitary descent of the implant, breast tissue, and inframammary fold.
- The medical term for breast lift is mastopexy.
- The goals of mastopexy are to reshape the breast, redistribute volume, and reposition the nipple-areola complex.
- The inframammary fold is a coalescence of thickened tissue from the skin and subcutaneous tissues to the periosteum.
- Tension on the wound increases when an implant is added to a mastopexy.
- The most common complications in breast lift are associated with circumareolar and inverted-T techniques.

Notes:

Why is it important to know about the different complications and issues with breast implants when working with clients after breast surgery?

Breast Reconstruction after Cancer

Why do people have reconstructive surgery after breast cancer? Cooper et al. state that "many patients seek reconstruction to reestablish breast shape and volume in an effort to limit the adverse biopsychosocial impact of mastectomy. Breast reconstruction can aid in restoring a patient's body image and sense of femininity as well as improving her overall quality of life" (Cooper et al., 2021).

What are some methods for reconstruction after treatment for breast cancer? According to BreastCancer.org, "there are two main breast reconstruction techniques: flap reconstruction and implant reconstruction." Flap reconstruction uses a flap of tissue from elsewhere in the client's body to reconstruct the breast shape and "also may include an implant (hybrid reconstruction). Implant reconstruction uses an implant — a silicon shell that's filled with silicone gel or saline (salt water) — to recreate the breast" (DePolo, 2023).

Many clients I see for breast reconstruction after breast cancer have reconstruction involving liposuction and fat transfer to the breast. Gabriel et al. states that "fat can be harvested from a number of sites, including the abdomen; medial, lateral, or anterior thighs; trochanteric region; flank; lower back, and knees." The fat is placed "between the overlying breast skin and the pectoralis major muscle" in a "postmastectomy reconstructed breast where host subcutaneous tissue has been voided." Fat transfer can reduce radiation-induced fibrosis, "but prior irradiation is also an important variable that could impact graft retention" (Gabriel et al., 2015a).

When does the surgery happen in the client's breast cancer journey? Citgez et al. states the "breast reconstruction methods after mastectomy include autologous or implant-based breast reconstructions, which can be performed at the same time as the breast cancer surgery (immediate reconstruction) or at a later time (delayed reconstruction)" (Citgez et al., 2020).

Mastectomy

Breast cancer-related surgeries include mastectomy, which is a surgical operation that removes all or part of the breast. According to Citgez et al., mastectomies "are classified into three types, namely, skin-sparing mastectomy (SSM), skin reduction mastectomy (SRM) and nipple-sparing mastectomy (NSM), which allow immediate reconstruction and require selection of specific incision" (Citgez et al., 2020).

- Skin-sparing mastectomy aims for the complete removal of the breast tissue, areola, and nipple while preserving the skin of the breast" (Citgez et al., 2020).
- Nipple-sparing mastectomy includes resection of the entire breast parenchyma while preserving the dermis and epidermis of the NAC. Nipple-sparing mastectomy is a safe technique in patients with small/medium breast size and low-grade ptosis without NAC invasion" (Citgez et al., 2020).
- Skin reduction mastectomy is applied to remove excess skin in patients with large or ptotic breasts" (Citgez et al., 2020).

Reconstruction

What is implant-based reconstruction? Clients may have breast implants as a part of reconstructing their breast after a diagnosis of breast cancer and mastectomy to remove the tumor. Dion et al. state that reconstructive options include "prosthetic devices (e.g., saline implants, silicone implants, tissue expanders) and autologous reconstruction methods using tissue flaps from adjoining or distant donor sites. Tissue flaps harvested from the lower abdomen—with skin, fat, and, occasionally, muscle—to create a breast mound are most commonly used for autologous breast reconstruction" (Dion et al., 2016). According to my experience, postoperative massage for the donor site after autologous reconstruction methods using a flap from the abdomen is like postoperative massage for an abdominoplasty on a client with a cancer history.

Citgez et al. state that "implant-based reconstruction can be done in one-stage (direct-to-implant) or two-stage (tissue expander followed by a permanent implant). The one-stage option has been improved by the diffusion of synthetic meshes and acellular dermal matrices (ADMs), which can be used to enlarge the sub-muscular pocket or to cover the implant above the muscle. The implant could be placed under or over the pectoralis major muscle" (Citgez et al., 2020). Graziano et al. found that "implant-based reconstruction is the most common method of immediate breast reconstruction in the United States, with acellular dermal matrices (ADMs) playing a significant role in implant support and coverage" and "in 39,800 immediate breast reconstructions, ADMs were used in 55.5% of cases" (Graziano et al., 2024).

Flores et al. state that "as an inert material, the implant's surface attracts lymphatic cells (T cells, macrophages) in an attempt at shielding the body against the foreign material, but without further inflammatory responses" and that "mainly breast cancer patients had implant-based complications when implants were contaminated. This shifted distribution raises the question of to what extent conservative breast cancer therapy alters immunologic processes." They state that "we do not know how the skin's microbiome in cancer patients behaves and what effects it has on the cellular immune response" (Flores et al., 2024).

Cazzato et al. found that "more than 50% of breast reconstructions involve a two-stage approach, in which a tissue expander (TE) is positioned under the pectoralis major muscle first and then it is replaced by a definitive implant when an adequate expansion is achieved (6 months on average)" (Cazzato et al., 2023).

In the last decade, prepectoral breast reconstruction has gained more and more popularity. Kim et al. conducted a systematic review and meta-analysis of prepectoral (PBR) versus subpectoral (SBR) breast reconstruction and found that "PBR considerably improved postoperative pain, BREAST-Q score, and upper arm function compared with SBR. Among postmastectomy radiation therapy patients, the incidence rates of capsular contracture were significantly lower in the PBR group than in the SBR group" (Y.H. Kim et al., 2024). Cazzato et al. state that "prepectoral breast reconstruction (PPBR) is usually regarded as the placement of an implant above the pectoralis major muscle in association with an acellular dermal matrix (ADM) that covers it completely. The presence of an ADM is essential, given its protective effect against capsular contracture onset" (Cazzato et al., 2023).

Notes:

What has your experience been with mastectomy reconstruction?

Acellular Dermal Matrix (ADM) Products

According to the FDA, "Acellular Dermal Matrix (ADM), a type of surgical mesh, is developed from human skin (such as FlexHD, AlloMax, AlloDerm) or animal skin (such as SurgiMend), in which the cells are removed, and the support structure is left in place." It's important to know that the FDA states that "although ADM is used for other types of reconstruction, the FDA has not cleared or approved ADM for use in breast reconstruction." The Mastectomy Reconstruction Outcomes Consortium (MROC) study data "showed significantly higher major complication rates of explantation, reoperation, and infections in patients with FlexHD and AlloMax brands of ADM two years after surgery, when compared to patients who received SurgiMend or AlloDerm brands, or no ADM" (Acellular Dermal Matrix (ADM) Products Used in Implant-Based Breast Reconstruction Differ in Complication Rates, 2021).

Silverstein & Momen conducted a retrospective analysis of 78 breast implants in 39 patients who underwent hybrid breast reconstruction and found that "polyglactin mesh and ADM were used in 24 breasts and 54 breasts, respectively. Implant malposition and capsular contracture occurred more frequently in the polyglactin cohort leading to 10 (41.7 percent) instances of re-operation for implant replacement compared to only 1 (1.9 percent) in the ADM cohort" (Silverstein & Momen, 2024).

Wound Healing and Complications

Where the incision is made has an effect on wound healing. Citgez et al. found that "incisions close to the edge of the pectoralis major muscle tolerate pressure better. On the other hand, incisions close to the lateral and inferior borders of the breast have a greater pressure load and cause delayed wound healing" (Citgez et al., 2020).

Radiotherapy (RT) can have an effect on surgery results. Citgez et al. found that "immediate breast reconstruction with implant ... is associated with a higher risk of capsular contracture after RT and an increased risk of implant loss in those with axillary lymph node dissection. In addition, there is a higher risk of complications compared to reconstruction with autologous tissue. The advantages of two-stage tissue-expander breast reconstruction include removal of irradiated tissue, correction of breast asymmetry, and better cosmetic outcomes in patients receiving RT. On the other hand, complication rates accounted for most cases undergoing two-stage reconstruction are higher than one-stage reconstruction with autologous tissue or implants (Citgez et al., 2020).

Another complication that occurs is animation deformity, which Citgez et al. state "can be observed in patients undergoing subpectoral implant-based breast reconstruction. It is usually corrected by a pocket change to the subcutaneous position or selective nerve ablation with botox injections" (Citgez et al., 2020).

A systematic review by Larsen et al. found that "studies investigating capsules affected by radiotherapy found a more pronounced inflammatory response and the capsules were generally thicker and fibrotic compared with nonirradiated capsules" (Larsen et al., 2021).

Radiation, Neurotoxin, and Capsular Contracture

Sobti et al. found that "capsular contracture is a common adverse outcome following implant breast reconstruction, often associated with radiation treatment." They propose that "muscle fibrosis from radiation treatment is the main contributor to breast contracture and asymmetry, thus treatment of post-radiation breast contracture should address the muscle specifically" (Sobti et al., 2020).

Capsular contracture may be an inaccurate term when the client has breast deformity after radiation. Sobti et al. found that the breast changes when the patient is under anesthesia. They found that "when subpectoral patients present with breast contracture, chemoparalysis of the muscle alone can resolve breast asymmetry, corroborating that muscle is a key contributor to breast contracture." They propose that "in the breast reconstruction patient population after radiation, the clinical diagnosis of *capsular* contracture is an inaccurate term to describe the breast contracture, as muscle fibrosis (not capsule) is the dominant contributing pathogenic factor" (Sobti et al., 2020).

According to Sobti et al., different changes in the breast as a result of post-mastectomy radiation therapy include "superolateral displacement of nipple-areolar complex, dimpling or creasing of the soft tissue envelope at the level of the pectoralis major muscle, flattening of inferior pole projection, and axillary fold crease" (Sobti et al., 2020).

Neurotoxin for Contracture

We just read that animation deformity can be reduced by Botox injections. Let's learn about some other uses of Botulinum toxin type A during breast cancer reconstruction. La Fleur et al. state that Botulinum toxin type A "is a neurotoxin that inhibits the release of the neurotransmitter acetylcholine at the neuromuscular junction with a goal to reduce excessive contraction of the target muscle" (la Fleur et al., 2020).

Neurotoxin has been used in several ways to reduce negative symptoms of breast reconstruction.

Gabriel et al. state that "tissue expander-based breast reconstruction has been plagued with pain and discomfort" and found that "infiltration of the pectoralis major muscle with neurotoxin in immediate, expander-based reconstruction may be beneficial in reducing pain and expediting expansions" (Gabriel et al., 2015b).

Zikiryakhodzhaev et al. share that a patient in Russia underwent subcutaneous mastectomy with immediate prepectoral breast reconstruction, then over the next few months experienced a persistent seroma, then firmness, then "a marked contour deformity of the reconstructed breast, and shape asymmetry. The reconstructed breast was painful to palpation. The clinical picture thus corresponded to Baker grade IV capsular contracture" with a pain level of 8. The patient was treated with incobotulinumtoxin A: "25 U into the area of the surgical scar, 20 U into the anterior leaf of the capsule, along the upper pole, and 25 U into the pectoralis major insertion." Complete pain relief was achieved within a week after the first injection. "At the follow-up visit 11 days later, improvement of the contracture was noted: the appearance of the scar reduced, and the capsule softened." A second round of Botulism Toxin type A was injected 11 days later, and "1 week after second injection, the patient had pronounced improvement in symptoms, specifically, the general shape of the reconstructed breast" (Zikiryakhodzhaev et al., 2021).

Figus et al. selected 13 patients who had "discomforting signs and symptoms from muscle contraction in the reconstructed breast" after "delayed unilateral breast reconstructions with LD flap and sub-pectoral implant after mastectomy." Patients were treated with Botulinum toxin A (BTX-A) percutaneous local injections, and "all patients reported a decrease or disappearance of the signs and symptoms. After 12 months, 11 patients received three BTX-A infiltrations, demonstrating considerable improvements compared to the pre-treatment status" (Figus et al., 2009).

Double check with the surgeon to confirm when massage is indicated after injection of Incobotulinumtoxin A. The Mayo Clinic advises not massaging the area for 24 hours after injection (Botox Injections, 2023).

Extrusion

Extrusion is a complication of breast implant surgery where the implant comes through the skin due to poor tissue coverage. Gargano et al. state that "breast surgery with implants requires good tissue coverage, especially in cases in which adjunctive radiation therapy has been used. Wound complication, such as dehiscence, infection, and fistulas, and clinically significant capsular contracture have been well reported in irradiated breast tissue. The irregular surface of the implant, the location of the pocket, and the pressure exerted by the implant against the skin can also lead to implant extrusion" (Gargano et al., 2009).

After they remove the implant, surgeons may use a flap of the client's skin from elsewhere on the body to add skin to the breast. In one study, Gargano et al. found that "complete correction of the extruded implants was achieved with the use of capsular flaps in all patients treated. Temporary skin depressions were seen in the acute phase of healing due, in part, to wound contracture and negative pressure of the suction drains. Both skin retractions and irregularities disappeared completely at 6 months" (Gargano et al., 2009).

Complications of Breast Reconstruction Using Liposuction and Fat Transfer to the Breast

According to the website Reclaim Your Curves, one potential negative side effect of autologous fat transfer is that "some of the fat injected into the breast area may die, which is called "necrosis." Symptoms of necrosis may include pain and bleeding, the skin turning dark blue or black, numbness, fever, and sores that ooze a bad-smelling discharge or pus" (Fat Grafting and Lipofilling, 2024). Have your client notify their surgeon immediately if they mention any of these signs and symptoms.

Other side effects or complications:

According to the International Expert Panel Consensus on Fat Grafting of the Breast, "potential complications of autologous fat grafting include fat necrosis, calcifications, and oil cyst formation" (Nava et al., 2019). According to the article 'Autologous fat grafting: Harvesting techniques,' complications may include "donor-site morbidity, like hematoma or, more frequently, local deformities caused by liposuction" (Fontes et al., 2018).

Don't let these complications scare you away from helping clients! According to the International Expert Panel Consensus on Fat Grafting of the Breast, "the majority of panelists consider fat grafting a safe procedure after breast-conserving surgery (69%) and mastectomy (86%) for breast cancer treatment. Fat grafting was also considered safe in patients with the BRCA mutation (71%), as long as adequate postoperative follow-up is maintained" (Nava et al., 2019).

Bottom Line:

- Breast reconstruction methods after mastectomy include autologous or implant-based breast reconstructions.
- Mastectomies are classified into three types, namely, skin-sparing mastectomy (SSM), skin reduction mastectomy (SRM), and nipple-sparing mastectomy (NSM).
- Implant-based reconstruction can be done in one-stage (direct-to-implant) or two-stage (tissue expander followed by a permanent implant).
- Immediate breast reconstruction with an implant may have a higher risk of capsular contracture after radiation therapy.
- Acellular Dermal Matrix (ADM), a type of surgical mesh, is developed from human or animal skin in which the cells are removed, and the support structure is left in place.
- Though it is often used "off-label," the FDA has not cleared or approved ADM for use in breast reconstruction.
- Animation deformity may happen in subpectoral implant-based breast reconstruction.
- Incisions close to the lateral and inferior borders of the breast have a greater pressure load and cause delayed wound healing.
- Capsules affected by radiotherapy may have a more pronounced inflammatory response.
- What looks like capsular contracture after radiation may actually be due to muscle fibrosis.
- Incobotulinumtoxin A may be used to treat capsular contracture.
- Extrusion is a complication of breast implant surgery where the implant comes through the skin due to poor tissue coverage.

- Complications of autologous fat grafting include fat necrosis, calcifications, and oil cyst formation.
- Radiation may cause superolateral displacement of the nipple-areolar complex, dimpling or creasing of the soft tissue envelope at the level of the pectoralis major muscle, flattening of inferior pole projection, and axillary fold crease.

Notes:

What would you say to an oncology massage client that asked you if they could see you for postoperative massage after breast implant related surgery?

Notes:

Gender-affirming surgery (GAS)

Gender Affirming Surgery Utilizing Breast Implants

An important note: I will be quoting research by experts in gender-affirming surgeries. These experts each use slightly different identity language. When I refer to patients receiving GAS, I include both transgender women and nonbinary people.

"Gender-affirming procedures are critical steps in helping transgender patients reach identity actualization and maximal quality of life" (Bekeny et al., 2020).

Treatment for gender dysphoria is the most common reason that transfeminine people seek gender-affirming breast augmentation surgery. According to Van Boerum et al., gender dysphoria "refers to the significant distress that results from an incongruence between the sex assigned at birth and the individual's gender identity. Social transition, hormones and gender-affirming surgeries (GAS) can be effective in the medical treatment of gender dysphoria. Transgender and gender non-binary individuals may choose to undergo one or more surgical procedures depending on their individual goals" (Van Boerum et al., 2019).

People of all genders can have breast implants. Transfeminine people get breast implant surgery to help them achieve a more feminine figure. Bekeny et al. state that "breast augmentation is an important and sometimes singular step in affirming a transfeminine individual's identity" (Bekeny et al., 2020).

Hormone therapy is advised before gender-affirming breast implant surgery in order for the patient to achieve as much natural breast growth as possible prior to augmentation. According to Van Boerum et al., "for transfeminine individuals, some breast growth can be achieved with the use of estrogen over the course of 1–2 years, but many still require breast augmentation for breasts that are proportionate to their frame" (Van Boerum et al., 2019).

Special Considerations for Transgender and Nonbinary Clients

If we are going to work with this underserved population it's important to know that, according to Bekeny et al., "transgender patients face contrasting rates of stigma, sexual abuse, physical assault, and lethal violence when compared to cisgendered peers. In healthcare, transgender patients report higher rates of ill-informed, unsupportive and even hostile caregivers." Bekeny et al. recommend that "by gaining insight into the specialized care of transgender patients, providers will start to bridge the gap and provide equitable service to all patients" (Bekeny et al., 2020).

What can we do to help transgender and nonbinary clients? Bekeny et al. state that "the patient's gender identity must be affirmed" and stress the importance of inquiring upfront about, consistently using, and properly documenting the patient's correct pronouns and chosen name. Bekeny et al. also note about language that "patients may refer to breast augmentation as "top surgery," and it is also important to acknowledge and document a patient's preferred way of speaking about their procedure" (Bekeny et al., 2020).

Frances Reed offers NCBTMB CE classes for massage therapists on Serving Transgender Clients in Holistic Health. Find more information at https://francesreed.com/training/.

What is the Postoperative Protocol?

Bekeny et al. state that "appropriate short-term care involves proper brasserie fitting and implant massage to soften the skin envelop. Activity restrictions vary across institutions, but it is generally recommended that patients avoid lifting more than five pounds and high-impact activities for a minimum of 4–6 weeks post-operatively" (Bekeny et al., 2020).

Chatterjee & Khanna, two surgeons who performed gender-affirming breast implant surgery in India, reviewed their protocols for a hundred and eleven patients of breast augmentation in trans women. The surgeons used "periareolar or inframammary" incisions, and the implants were placed "in a subfascial pocket." Patients had a postoperative protocol of "restricted shoulder movements for 3 weeks, use of an inner brassiere and outer sports vest for 2 months" and "from 3 weeks postoperatively, routine massage of breasts for a period of 6 to 8 weeks were advised" (Chatterjee & Khanna, 2020).

Chatterjee & Khanna stated that "patients are taught massage of the breasts which is started 3 weeks after the operation in sequence of upward, downward, medial, and lateral firm pressure and circular motion with both hands in clockwise and anticlockwise manner for at least 20 minutes twice daily for a period of 6 weeks. In addition, patients are asked to lie prone for about two hours a day even if not at a stretch" (Chatterjee & Khanna, 2020).

Chatterjee & Khanna found that "capsular contracture meriting operative intervention occurred only in two patients but one of them refused operation" (Chatterjee & Khanna, 2020).

What are Complications to Watch Out for in the Transgender and Nonbinary Population?

Bekeny et al. state that "the most common complications specific to breast implantation in both the cisgender and transgender populations include symmastia, capsular contracture, reduced breast or nipple sensation, implant leakage, or implant migration" (Bekeny et al., 2020).

The good news is that capsular contracture rates are lower in the transgender and nonbinary populations. Schoffer et al. state that "estrogen exposure seems to be the first possible reason for a lower rate of capsular contracture" in gender-affirming breast augmentation surgery (Schoffer et al., 2022).

Exercise after surgery can affect breast implants. Bekeny et al. state that "pectoralis major hypertrophy can lead to progressive lateralization of the implant over-time, so this should be monitored for in patients with subpectoral implants" (Bekeny et al., 2020). This lateralization of the implant is distressing to many transgender clients.

Symmastia

Let's learn more about symmastia. Zingaretti et al. state that "symmastia, the medial confluence of the breast tissue across the midline, is occasionally encountered in clinical practice, but relatively uncommon. In observations, this condition presents itself as a web of skin, fat, and tissue merged together, resulting in a reduction of the intermammary sulcus... Acquired symmastia is fairly common, and it's usually a consequence of bilateral breast augmentation, whereby overaggressive dissection of the medial aspect of the implant pocket produces a communication of both implant pockets across the midline" (Zingaretti et al., 2018).

Kalaria et al. performed a retrospective chart review of 23 iatrogenic symmastia patients and stated that "symmastia is most often caused by pectoralis major sternal dehiscence during subpectoral breast augmentation. In the senior author's experience, all patients with iatrogenic symmastia previously had a submuscular breast augmentation. The ASAPS survey supports multiple causes for symmastia with retromuscular breast augmentation occurring in the majority of patients. Repair of symmastia should include securing Scarpa's fascia to the sternum, reattaching the pectoralis major to the sternum, avoiding another subpectoral implant, and using postoperative modalities to protect the repair" (Kalaria et al., 2019). ASAPS stands for American Society for Aesthetic Plastic Surgery.

Notes:

Sketch an image showing the difference between lateralization of a breast implant and symmastia.

What Other Operations Can Be Combined with Breast Implants?

Van Boerum et al. state that "liposuction and fat grafting are common cosmetic procedures that can be used to improve body contour in transmasculine, transfeminine, and non-binary individuals" (Van Boerum et al., 2019). Changes to the contours of hips, butt, flanks, and belly are the most common for transfeminine patients. Fat grafting "will typically result in 50–60% permanent take of the graft, and can be performed a number of times for optimal results" (Van Boerum et al., 2019). We will learn more about fat grafting later in the class.

Bottom Line:

- Gender dysphoria describes the significant distress that results from an incongruence between the sex assigned at birth and the individual's gender identity.
- When working with transgender clients, gender identity must be affirmed, which includes inquiring about the client's pronouns and chosen name.
- Pectoralis major hypertrophy can lead to progressive lateralization of the implant over time.
- Symmastia is the medial confluence of the breast tissue across the midline.
- Liposuction and fat grafting can be used to improve body contour in transmasculine, transfeminine, and non-binary individuals.

Notes:

What would you say to a plastic surgeon that asked you why they should refer their gender affirming surgery clients to you for postoperative massage after breast implant related surgery?

Define in your own words, the following terms. What would you say to a client that asked about each condition?

Animation deformity

Bottoming out

Double bubble

Calcium deposit

Capsular contracture

Extrusion

Hematoma

Rippling

Rupture

Seroma

Slide-down deformity

Symmastia

Massage after Breast Implant Surgery

I'm always surprised when surgeons don't mention professional massage sessions to their clients after breast surgery. Self-massage of smooth (not textured) breast implants is a part of many plastic surgeons' postoperative protocol, and many clients are hesitant or unsure of how to best self-massage. Booking a professional massage session gives the clients a chance to feel the pressure and speed of the massage, and they often leave with more confidence in their ability to self-massage. Let's look at research on self-massage protocols (in the online class, I share the specific 30- and 60-minute protocols I use with my clients).

Surgeons often advise their patients to perform self-massage after getting breast implants. Over a thousand plastic surgeons responded to an ASPS member survey on common practices in breast augmentation, and researchers found that "postoperative massage is still popular with over half of respondents" (Sinno & Hidalgo, 2016). ASPS is the American Society of Plastic Surgeons.

Surgeons have been incorporating MLD into postoperative care for breast implant surgery for over a dozen years. The 'Cosmetic Bootcamp Primer: Comprehensive Aesthetic Management' states that "manual lymphatic drainage and capsule massage are employed to accelerate resolution of tissue edema which will presumably minimize early capsular contracture. A recent multi-center study revealed complication rates significantly lower than published data" (Beer et al., 2011, pg. 213).

Are some surgeons not recommending professional massage because moving the tissue too soon after a breast implant is dangerous? Sood et al. did a literature review on patient self-massage techniques and found that short bouts of self-massage were often not enough to reduce capsular contracture rates, but they did not increase the percentage of capsular contracture. The intention of the massage is to press the surrounding breast tissue firmly against the capsule. (Sood et al., 2017).

- Two studies had patients start massage two weeks postoperatively and found no difference in massage vs. control (Sood et al., 2017).
- Two other studies started massage two or three days after surgery, and the results were either no capsular contracture or 8% of patients experiencing mild capsular contracture (Sood et al., 2017).
- The study that resulted in 0% capsular contracture had a protocol of "exercises were performed in the supine position, with multiple clockwise maneuvers exerting as much force as tolerated, for 5 minutes per breast, twice daily" force applied was measured from 80 - 300 mm hg (Sood et al., 2017). In contrast, my usual MLD pressure is under 20 mm hg.

When I speak to a surgeon about the timing of postoperative massages, I ask them when they are recommending their patients start self-massage. Therapists can certainly design a 30-minute session that can incorporate MLD and the same self-massage techniques that surgeons are recommending postoperatively.

Notes:

Take a look at the 30 minute protocol shown in the online class.

List and describe the elements of the protocol. Why is each section important to the massage? How does each section help the client after breast implant surgery?

Notes:

What would you say to a plastic surgeon that asked you why they should send their patients to you for postoperative massage after breast implant related surgery?

Notes:

Why do Clients Book a Massage After Breast Implant Surgery?

In my experience, most cosmetic clients are afraid of complications from the surgery, worried that the implants will not drop, and hesitant to perform self-breast massage. Massage after breast implant surgery can include:

- Pain-relieving Swedish massage strokes on the neck, shoulders, and back,
- Manual lymphatic drainage to reduce swelling of the breasts and liposuctioned areas,
- Instruction on self-massage so the client can feel breast massage and learn self-breast massage from the therapist and
- Scar massage on breast implant /breast lift scars in the proliferative and maturation stage of healing.

Guenter Klose, one of my teachers and an expert in the treatment of lymphedema, says "postsurgical clients who can benefit from manual lymph drainage include those recovering from cosmetic surgeries such as face-lifts, breast augmentation, and liposuction and orthopedic surgeries such as joint repair or replacement. Manual lymph drainage effectively reduces swelling even before appropriate muscle movement and function can be restored" (2014). Often, a surgeon will only allow very light exercise in the weeks after surgery. Manual Lymphatic Drainage massage can help reduce swelling before patients are allowed to use exercise and joint movement to help their lymphatic system.

MLD After Surgery to Reduce Stress and Pain

MLD has been found to reduce stress after breast cancer surgery. In a study by Ko, 12 participants received a 20-minute MLD session after breast cancer surgery five times per week for four weeks. The results showed that MLD is "an effective method in reducing stress and pain in patients with postoperative breast cancer" (Ko, 2021).

Why Might MLD Reduce Stress and Pain?

MLD can reduce stress in healthy subjects, which can be measured through heart rate variability (HRV). Kim et al. found that a 40-minute MLD session is "highly effective in increasing HRV and cardiac parasympathetic activity in normal subjects" (Kim et al., 2009).

Keser & Esmer have also found that MLD may have an effect on the experience of pain. They measured participants' pain levels before and after an MLD session and found that "MLD increases pain threshold and pain tolerance significantly in healthy subjects." They explained that rhythmic stimuli like MLD may create "inhibitions on the nociceptive receptors of the skin" (Keser & Esmer, 2019).

Pleasant Touch to Reduce Pain

Massage therapists can also deliver a gentle, dynamic touch called 'pleasant touch' or 'CT touch.' Fusaro et al. have found that "pleasant touch can successfully reduce experimentally induced pain" and "when people experience pain under normal circumstances, gently touching the aching area usually results in physical and emotional relief." Pleasant touch involves C tactile (CT) receptors (Fusaro et al., 2022).

Fusaro et al. state that:

- "CT-afferents, found in particular in the hairy skin, react mainly when stroked at a particular velocity of 3–6 cm/s" (Fusaro et al., 2022),
- Applied force ... between 0.04 and 5 millinewton is required to activate CT-receptors" (Fusaro et al., 2022),
- "Touch at skin-temperature seems to be optimal to elicit the firing of CT-fibers while warm and cool touches activate them to a lesser extent" (Fusaro et al., 2022), and
- "The firing of these CT afferents is coupled with a subjective sensation of pleasantness" (Fusaro et al., 2022).

The keys to this touch are a combination of slow, gentle indentation and motion to hairy skin. Clients often are hesitant to touch or massage themselves, and loved ones may stop touching the client after surgery for fear of hurting them. **Their time with a well-trained massage therapist may be the only time our clients feel comfortable enough to receive touch in the weeks after their surgery.**

Notes:

What has your experience been with using MLD on clients after surgery?

What about pleasant touch?

Surgeon Protocol for Postoperative Massage After Breast Implant Surgery

Giometti et al. reviewed data from 100 women who received breast implants. 30 received anatomic implants, and 70 received round implants and surgeries had only "4 cases of grade III and IV capsular contracture, which is more common with the use of round implants." The surgeon "routinely prescribed oral montelukast 10 mg for 3 months together with vitamin E at a daily dose of 800 IU, as a protocol for the prevention of capsular contracture. Manual lymphatic drainage commences on the fifth postoperative day, and is performed 2 to 3 times per week, for a month on average. The use of a compression bra is started in the immediate postoperative period and maintained for 30 days" (Giometti et al., 2016).

Protocol for Implant-based Breast Reconstruction

There is no common oncology massage protocol for helping clients after implant-based breast reconstruction who have no surgical complications.

Nevola et al. found that "the use of massage therapy techniques ... and manual lymphatic drainage are usual in the clinical practice, but there is a lack of protocols and studies that prove the efficacy in patients underwent oncological plastic surgery reconstruction with implants" (Nevola et al., 2014).

In 2018, Mazuquin et al. looked at the clinical practice of physical therapists for patients undergoing breast reconstruction for breast cancer in Brazil and the UK and found that "only half of women having breast reconstruction were routinely referred to physical therapy postoperatively." Physical therapists surveyed shared that "the main reasons for referral to physical therapy were for management of complications after surgery followed by referrals for patients with a history of shoulder problems before having a breast reconstruction" (Mazuquin et al., 2021).

How to Provide a Customized Massage After Breast Implant Surgery

Menard reminds us that "massage therapy, as defined by its practitioners, is a complex intervention that employs multiple modalities, incorporates therapeutic relationship and patient education as an essential aspect of the therapy, and is grounded in the biopsychosocial model, wherein clients are viewed as active participants in their own care rather than passive recipients" (Menard, 2015). We treat the whole person that comes into our office for massage, not just a breast that has had surgery.

We can provide a customized massage that addresses the client at their current level of healing by actively choosing which massage strokes to use and modifying our massage strokes and the session itself.

First, let's look at the massage strokes we might use to help clients after breast implant surgery. I commonly use Swedish massage strokes of effleurage, petrissage, and friction, as well as manual lymphatic drainage. We can also use compression, holding, and passive and active joint movement.

Massage Session After Surgery Vs. Typical Relaxation Massage Session

When comparing a massage session after surgery to a typical relaxation massage session, I can modify several aspects of the massage itself and the session protocol to make the experience safer for a client recovering from surgery. Modifications include:

- Working at a lighter pressure and shallower depth on the tissue,
- Increasing or reducing the broadness of my contact. Am I using just my fingertips or all of my fingers and the entire palm of my hand for the massage stroke? For example, using fingertips can be less invasive if pressure is light or more invasive if deeper pressure is used with a smaller focal point of massage,
- Matching the direction of my massage strokes with the direction of lymphatic flow versus strokes going in several directions over the length of the massage session,
- Decreasing the drag on tissues,
- Decreasing the speed of the massage strokes,
- Limiting client movement during the massage to diaphragmatic breathing,
- Keep a rhythm in massage strokes, as well as slow the rhythm down. I find that meditative music helps me to keep a slower pace,
- Modifying the overall protocol of the session by ensuring I have enough time for each aspect and not rushing through sections of the massage, and
- Moving slower around the client and using eye contact and a soft, soothing voice.

I consider how both the client's tissues and their nervous system would respond to each massage modification. As the client's healing proceeds from the inflammatory stage to the proliferation and maturation stage, I can change or reduce each of these modifications. For instance, a client in the maturation stage can tolerate:

- Deeper pressure and depth on the tissue,
- A more focal pressure with fingers and thumbs and a deeper compression and stroke using the whole hand,
- Massage strokes in all directions during the massage session,
- Strokes that place drag on tissues,
- Increased speed of the massage strokes,
- Incorporating client movement at the neck and shoulder joints,
- Faster rhythm in massage strokes and
- Upbeat conversation and cracking jokes.

The conversation with the plastic surgeon will often just cover the basics of the massage protocol. A fixed protocol manages the following:

- Location of massage intervention on the body (where are we massaging and where are we not massaging?),
- Frequency of massage sessions (how many sessions per week?),
- Duration of each massage session (how long is each session?) and
- Massage techniques that are off-limits (no deep tissue, no tapotement, no hydrotherapy).

Notes:

Take a look at the possible session modifications.

Describe why each modification is an important tool to have in our massage toolbox to help clients healing from surgery.

The value of a massage session starts at the intake interview. Kerr et al. state that "physical touch and face-to-face interaction, entailing eye gaze and retinal eye lock, are two types of contact that produce neurophysiological effects on the body." Making eye contact is an important part of my massage sessions. Kerr et al. have found that "when interacting with trusted others, a number of chemicals are released, including oxytocin and vasopressin, both of which help to lower the physiological stress response and aid growth and wound healing" (Kerr et al., 2019).

How Does Eye Contact Help Our Clients?

- "Eye gaze and retinal eye lock between an anxious person and a trusted "other" has a direct effect on the synchronization of the right brain hemispheres and the quietening of the sympathetic nervous system and amygdala, increasing the ability to deal with trauma" (Kerr et al., 2019).
- "This "eye contact effect" modulates activity in structures in the social brain network, aiding communicative intention and affective arousal" (Kerr et al., 2019).
- "There is growing evidence of the link between these neurophysiological reactions and a decreased level of morbidity and mortality through such changes as an increased capacity for hope, the capacity to reframe vulnerability and deal with trauma, and neurophysiological reactions related to the placebo effect" (Kerr et al., 2019).

Notes:

Let's revisit a writing prompt from earlier in class.

What would you say to a plastic surgeon that asked you why they should send their patients to you for postoperative massage after breast implant related surgery? Would you add any information we just covered in class to the conversation? Which studies might be valuable?

Notes:

Draping and Positioning

- If a client has had a fat transfer to the breast, I suggest that clients leave on their surgical bra if they like and drape them with a breast drape and/or the massage sheet.
- I ask all clients to begin by lying facing up underneath the sheet. I add a bolster when I re-enter the massage room. I lay a pillowcase over the breast area, then remove the sheet from underneath the breast drape to access the abdomen.
- If I am going to provide massage on the surgery area, I recommend clients remove any compression garments they are wearing that cover the area that had surgery. If it is a bra, it can be unhooked by the client during the massage if needed (so they don't have to completely remove and put it back on while under ROM restrictions of the shoulder and arms).
- Be sure to wipe the skin clean from any oil or lotion used before the client dons their garment again. Oils break down the elastic in compression garments.
- When I am performing breast massage, I undrape to the level previously agreed upon when the breast massage release form was signed.
- I ask clients how their surgeon recommended that they lie when sleeping and replicate that on the massage table using bolsters and wedges. If the client is especially anxious, I will elevate their legs above their heart using a leg wedge (Søndergaard, 2022).
- In the article 'Breast Reconstruction With a Flap: What to Expect at Home,' MyHealth.Alberta.ca recommends that clients "prop up the arm on the side of your surgery on a pillow when you sit or lie down. Try to keep your

arm above the level of your heart. This will help reduce swelling" (Breast Reconstruction With a Flap: What to Expect at Home, n.d.).

- It's also valuable to know what position the client's body had to be in during their treatment for cancer. Was their arm or body in a certain position during the surgery or radiation treatments? Be aware that resuming this position may bring up emotions for the client.

Notes:

Take a look at the protocols shown in the online class.

List and describe the elements of the protocol. Why is each section important to the massage? How does each section help the client after breast implant surgery?

Notes:

Stages of Wound Healing

I adjust the massage I offer based on where the client is in the stages of wound healing.

Hemostasis - cut to blood clot - body forms platelet plug with threads of fibrin, which are like a molecular binding agent.

Inflammatory - alongside Hemostasis - injured blood vessels leak transudate (made of water, salt, and protein), causing localized swelling. Inflammation controls bleeding and prevents infection. Damaged cells, pathogens, and bacteria need to be removed. Inflammation is a natural part of the body's healing process.

Proliferative - rebuilding using new tissue made up of collagen and extracellular matrix.

Maturation - collagen is remodeled from type III to type I. Collagen is aligned along tension lines and water is reabsorbed.

What Types of Massage are Best at Each Stage of Wound Healing?

Hemostasis - we won't see clients this soon after surgery. I usually wait at least 4-5 days after surgery to massage the area of surgery. If the client wanted a soothing relaxation massage on unaffected areas like the neck, upper back, or feet, with surgeon approval, we could give it while the client is supine and in their compression garment. Slow, gentle strokes could give the same benefits that we read about in the earlier sections on massage, reducing pain and anxiety after surgery.

Inflammatory - Manual Lymphatic Drainage - we can help to reduce swelling. The client's macrophages are removing debris, and their lymphatic system is the sump pump of the body. If the client is experiencing soreness and/or reduced Range of Motion (ROM) in the neck and shoulders, massage techniques aimed at increasing comfort can be used according to the client's pain tolerance and surgeon's restrictions on shoulder movement. Know and respect the surgeon's restrictions on shoulder range of motion. Moving edema into the lymphatic system and reducing pain is the name of the game in the inflammatory stage. It's too soon for deeper work.

Proliferative/Maturation - Manual Lymphatic Drainage is still useful, and I use it before and after techniques to help increase shoulder ROM and remodel scar tissue.

In the proliferation stage, new tissues are forming, so load, pressure, stretch can still cause tenderness, even weeks into recovery. If the client has a flare up, it means the body has entered the inflammatory stage again.

It's not ideal to have prolonged symptoms of inflammation. Inflammation can cause pain, and pain can cause inflammation. General and systemic inflammation can also influence one another. Chronic inflammation is NOT useful to the body.

In his Medbridge class, 'Tissue Injury: Mechanisms of Inflammation and Repair,' Physical Therapist Andrew J. Opett states that contractures can occur during the proliferation stage of wound healing and stresses the importance of range of motion (ROM), stretching, and scar massage (Opett, n.d.).

Notes:

Label the different stages of wound healing on this image.

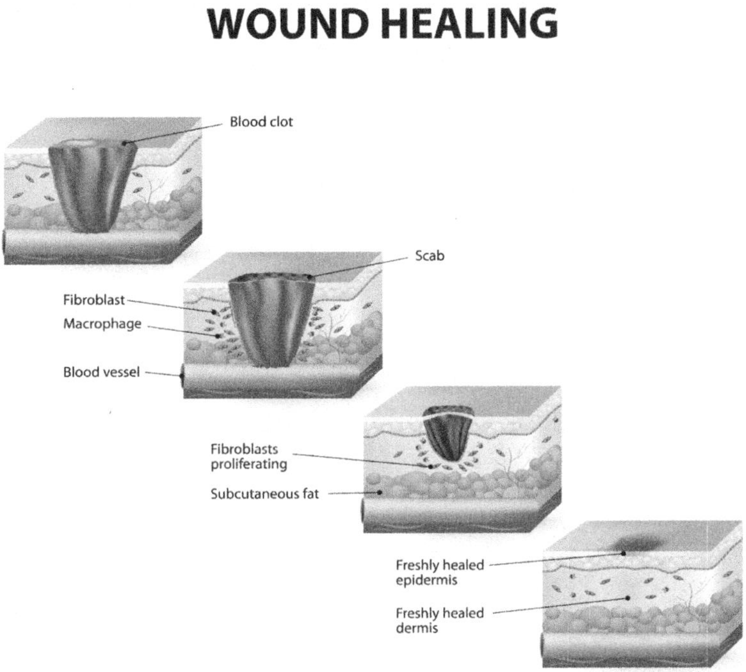

Notes:

Did you ever have a client who did "too much, too soon" after their plastic surgery and had a longer healing process as a result? Could the same thing happen if we did "too much, too soon" in our massage sessions?

Notes:

What We May Feel During the Massage After Breast Surgery

Jelly-like tissue consistency

If we are massaging edematous tissue, the tissue texture may sometimes feel rubbery or doughy. Belgrado et al. state that "the chronic lymphatic impairment leads to an accumulation of proteins, free water, and a form of jelly composed of water bound with hyaluronan" (Belgrado et al., 2023).

Mondors

Mondor's cording sometimes appears at the anterolateral thoracoabdominal wall below the breast after surgery. Amano & Shimizu state that "Mondor's disease (MD) occurs with palpable subcutaneous cord-like indurations beneath the skin. Usually, MD is a benign, self-limited disease that resolves spontaneously in four to eight weeks." Interestingly, these researchers state that "almost all MDs appeared to be thrombophlebitis of the superficial vein, while some cases occurred due to lymphangitis" and that axillary web syndrome is a form of Mondor's disease (Amano & Shimizu, 2018).

Palpable Granulomas

We may feel granulomas in the breast tissue. Elahi et al. state that "silicone "bleeding" has been described from both ruptured and intact implants and can induce local granulomas, resulting in typical macrophage invasion, giant cell formation, and eventual scarring or disseminated granulomatosis due to the component's high-fat solubility. They present as indurated, palpable granulomas found in cutaneous tissues, lymph nodes, and the breast. In rare cases, they may extend to the lungs, lower limbs, liver, and spleen" (Elahi et al., 2022).

What happens when silicone is put in the body? We can learn about the body's reaction to silicone by looking into what happens after a silicone injection. According to Harlim et al., when hydrophobic silicone is injected into the body, it "triggers adsorption of plasma proteins on the surface of silicone, and a "protein matrix" is formed. The latter triggers the immune system: blood clotting, fibrinolysis, and activation of kinin and complement systems. In addition, various cytokines, chemokines, and growth factors in the matrix on the silicone surface cause activation of certain immune cells." This inflammatory reaction "produces a microenvironment containing tumor necrosis factor (TNF) α, which in turn triggers maturation of extracellular matrix (ECM) proteins within fibroblasts, thereby causing fibrosis" (Harlim et al., 2018). Sometimes silicone is found in the lymphatic system. Harlim et al. state that smaller silicone "microdroplets of <15 μm may undergo further phagocytosis by macrophages and will be transported through lymphatic vessels. By contrast, large microdroplets cannot be phagocytosed, and ... the reaction between silicone and the tissue creates fibrous capsules and triggers granuloma formation" (Harlim et al., 2018).

Calcification

If inflammation or infection is present, calcification deposits can also form. These feel like "hard lumps under the skin around the implant" (Risks and complications of breast implants, 2023).

Enlarged lymph nodes

Silicone-related lymphadenopathies are rare and, according to Elahi et al., "consist of a deposition of silicone in one or more lymph nodes on the drainage path of the breast. An inflammatory reaction ensues, which may or may not be symptomatic over time. It may simply present as a palpable lump, which goes unnoticed until later detected as incidentalomas. They are most commonly found in the axillary regions but can also be found in the mediastinal, cervical, and internal mammary regions" (Elahi et al., 2022).

Notes:

Contraindications to Massage

The first two big contraindications to breast massage are the client's unwillingness to consent to massage and inability to give written consent. Make sure you have great communication with your client before beginning.

I use the same main contraindications with my post-plastic surgery massage modalities as I would if I were providing massage for a client with lymphedema.

Infection - I do not massage if they have an untreated infection. I ask clients to take antibiotics for a few days and have their plastic surgeon clear them for massage before I rebook them.

I do not provide any massage if the client has a fever. WoundSource has a great post on the signs of an infected wound. They include fever of over 101 degrees Fahrenheit, overall malaise, and redness, pain, swelling and unusual wound drainage color and smell (8 Signs of Wound Infection, 2016).

Pumps and Filters - I don't move lymphatic fluid or give any massage if the client has acute infection, cellulitis, suspected DVT / sudden below-knee swelling/shortness of breath, uncontrolled heart failure, or kidney failure.

When Can We NOT Help Clients

It's important to realize we are not experts in anything other than massage. When in doubt, refer out. If their surgeon is local, they can email or call their surgeon, the nurse, or the patient coordinator. If an out-of-town surgeon, have them inform the surgeon, then refer them to their primary care physician.

Notes:

What contraindications have you seen in your post-surgical massage clients? How did you handle the situation?

What information are clients receiving in their postoperative visits?

Notes:

List the most interesting topics that might be covered in our clients' visits with their plastic surgeon.

Bottom Line:

- Self-massage of smooth (not textured) breast implants is a part of many plastic surgeons' postoperative protocol.
- Postoperative massage is still popular, with over half of respondents surveyed using an ASPS survey.
- MLD can reduce edema, stress, and pain levels.
- Pleasant touch can successfully reduce experimentally induced pain.
- Stages of wound healing include Hemostasis, Inflammatory, Proliferative, and Maturation.
- Silicone "bleeding" has been described from both ruptured and intact implants and can induce local granulomas.
- Silicone-related lymphadenopathies consist of the deposition of silicone in one or more lymph nodes on the drainage path of the breast.
- Mondor's disease describes palpable subcutaneous cord-like indurations beneath the skin.
- Contraindications to massage include acute untreated infection, cellulitis, suspected DVT / sudden below-knee swelling / shortness of breath, fever, uncontrolled heart failure, and kidney failure.

Notes:

Define in your own words, the following terms. What would you say to a client that asked about each condition?

Animation deformity

Bottoming out

Double bubble

Calcium deposit

Capsular contracture

Extrusion

Hematoma

Mondors

Rippling

Rupture

Seroma

Slide-down deformity

Symmastia

Breast Implant Removal Without Replacement of implants

Why do people choose explant surgery?

Some clients have older breast implants, are tired of having breast implants or want a smaller breast and choose to have their breast implants removed without replacing them with another set of implants. Other clients believe their implants are making them sick and choose to have them removed without any replacement. Clients can choose to just have the implant removed or have the implant and capsule removed. Some clients have additional surgeries along with breast implant removal to change the shape of their breasts. They can also have a breast lift and/or liposuction and fat transfer to the breasts.

It's relatively simple to understand the client's motivation if they are having surgery to remove older breast implants or voluntarily taking steps to have smaller breasts. They will generally be happy with the results of their surgery if they choose a quality surgeon and have no complications after surgery.

In my experience, the client's journey is much more complicated and emotional if they are removing their implants because they fear that they have systematic symptoms associated with breast implants (SSBI), which they may call breast implant illness.

What may be happening if the client's implants are making them sick? First of all, It's important to know the difference between breast implant illness (BII) and BIA-ALCL:

What is BII?

The FDA reports that "symptoms such as fatigue, memory loss, rash, "brain fog," and joint pain may be associated with breast implants, and some patients and clinicians may use the term "breast implant illness" to describe these symptoms or use these terms when reporting them to the FDA. The top 10 most common symptoms reported to the FDA's medical device report database for patients with breast implants include fatigue (49 percent), brain fog (25 percent), joint pain (25 percent), anxiety (24 percent), hair loss (21 percent), depression (19 percent), rash (18 percent), autoimmune diseases (18 percent), inflammation (18 percent) and/or weight problems (18 percent)" (FDA Updates Analysis of Medical Device Reports of Breast Implant Illness and Breast Implant-Associated Lymphoma, 2020).

This is important to understand. Clients who have breast implant removal surgery because they suspect they have breast implant illness may be suffering from:

- fatigue,
- brain fog,
- joint pain,
- anxiety,
- depression,
- rash,
- autoimmune diseases, and/or
- inflammation.

Though I see so many posts and comments about people with BII experiencing a rapid reduction in symptoms after the removal of breast implants and capsules, massage therapists still need to prepare to provide support for clients who don't experience a quick 'miracle cure.'

- Helping clients with fatigue may mean scheduling the massage at the time they are least fatigued and/or offering in-home services.
- Brain fog may mean that clients need additional reminders for their massage sessions.
- We may see medication for anxiety, depression, and autoimmune diseases on their health history forms.
- We may see a chronic rash on the body during their massage session.
- They may complain of inflammation and joint pain.

Notes:

What is your experience with breast implant illness? Why do you think it happens?

What is BIA-ALCL?

Breast implant-associated anaplastic large cell lymphoma (BIA-ALCL) is a type of non-Hodgkin's lymphoma, which is a cancer of the immune system. This rare cancer is diagnosed with an exam, imaging, and testing.

Another breast implant complication is squamous cell carcinoma.

Squamous Cell Carcinoma

Very rarely, squamous cell carcinoma (SCC) can also grow in the scar tissue (capsule) that forms around breast implants.

What do people think may be causing BII?

There are several different names for the constellation of BII symptoms listed above by the FDA, including ASIA, BII, SSBI, and Siliconosis / Silicone Incompatibility Syndrome (SIS). There are also several different theories about its cause or causes. Let's look at a few possibilities.

Many people agree that BII may occur because of silicone-induced immune activation. Theories about the cause of BII include autoimmune syndrome, biofilm, and silicone toxicity. Some people also point a finger at heavy metals in the breast implant as a cause of symptoms.

Notes:

What insight did you find in the class articles and videos about breast implant illness and heavy metals?

Autoimmune/inflammatory syndrome induced by adjuvants (ASIA)

ASIA is a term used more commonly outside the USA to refer to the symptoms of BII. What is an adjuvant? Cohen Tervaert et al. state that "adjuvants are compounds that, when introduced into the body, enhance a specific immune reaction resulting in higher titers of antibodies, for instance against specific pathogens ... During the last decade, it became clear that implanted medical implants, including injectables such as silicones and polypropylene meshes, may act as adjuvants" (Cohen Tervaert et al., 2022).

Watad et al. believe that this condition starts when "exposure to an adjuvant leads to an aberrant autoimmune response." The researchers examined 300 cases from the ASIA syndrome registry and found that "the mean age at disease onset was 37 years, and the mean duration of time latency between adjuvant stimuli and development of autoimmune conditions was 16.8 months, ranging between 3 days to 5 years. Arthralgia, myalgia, and chronic fatigue were the most frequently reported symptoms. Eighty-nine percent of patients were also diagnosed with another defined rheumatic/autoimmune condition. The most frequent autoimmune disease related to ASIA syndrome was undifferentiated connective tissue disease (UCTD). ASIA syndrome is associated with a high incidence of UCTD and positive anti-nuclear antibodies (ANA) test" (Watad et al., 2018).

The term Breast Implant Illness is common in the United States of America. Cohen Tervaert et al. state that "'adjuvant hypothesis' explains BII. Therefore, one should use the term 'ASIA (autoimmune/autoinflammatory syndrome induced by adjuvants) due to silicone incompatibility syndrome' rather than the nonspecific term 'BII' for this syndrome" (Cohen Tervaert et al., 2022).

Silicone migration and silicone-associated lymphadenopathy

Silicone from breast implants can travel to other parts of the body. A study at the Mayo Clinic by McConnell et al. examined 162 tissue samples from 72 patients "during augmentation, capsulectomy with or without replacement mammoplasty, mastectomy, or biopsy procedures." The tissue samples were tested for silicon, and the researchers found that "tissue silicon levels (breast parenchymal and periprosthetic capsular tissue) in patients with silicone gel implants were much higher than in patients with saline implants or nonaugmented breasts" (McConnell et al., 1997).

Rajgor et al. state that "silicone-associated lymphadenopathy occurs following migration of silicone particles to regional lymph nodes. This can be a consequence of implant rupture or when microscopic amounts of silicone gel leak from the outer shell (known as 'gel bleed'). The majority of cases result in axillary or mediastinal lymphadenopathy" (Rajgor et al., 2021).

The silicone shell of a saline implant can also pose a problem. A case report by Rajgor et al. shared details of a patient with "multiple palpable cervical lymph nodes bilaterally in levels IV and Vb," and an ultrasound showed "multiple lymph nodes with the snowstorm sign." The core biopsy "confirmed a silicone granuloma (siliconoma) ... likely caused by bleeding gel from the silicone shell of her saline-based implants." The patient's implants had not ruptured (Rajgor et al., 2021).

We learned earlier that a snowstorm sign is when silicone gel droplets mixed with breast tissue create a "heterogeneous echogenic pattern and dispersion of the ultrasound beam causing posterior acoustic shadowing" (Rajgor et al., 2021).

Notes:

Have you had clients that suffered from silicone-related issues? What treatments did they try?

Do Some Types of Implants Cause More Symptoms than Others?

Katsnelson et al. reviewed 248 patients with symptoms attributed to BII who underwent breast implant removal with capsulectomy and found that "there is an underlying inflammatory response associated with the implant capsule, a response which appears to be more common in silicone versus saline and textured versus smooth implants. This response may be associated with symptoms of BII" (Katsnelson et al., 2020). Flores et al. state that "the uneven surface of textured implants offers more possibilities for pathogens to settle and evade the immune system, despite meticulous antisepsis, therefore possibly resulting in an increase of unnoticed implant contamination and subclinical infection rates leading to implant damage" (Flores et al., 2024). We will likely not see many clients with textured implants because postoperative massage is not recommended for clients with textured implants.

Biofilm

Biofilms may also play a role in symptoms that clients with breast implants experience. Yang et al. state that biofilms are "microbial communities bound to the surfaces of living tissues, implants, and medical devices. Infections caused by biofilms are difficult to eliminate and result in persistent and chronic and most likely low-grade inflammation reactions. Several studies show a correlation between the presence of microbial biofilms on various medical implants and persistent inflammation in surrounding tissue" (Yang et al., 2022).

Lee et al. evaluated 50 consecutive patients, self-referring for explantation due to BII, and found "comparison of BII and control groups revealed key histopathological and microbiological differences. The BII group had a 50% higher rate of synoviocyte metaplasia than that of controls ... Additionally, the BII group had a 6-fold greater rate of positive cultures, with the most prominent organism being *Propionibacterium acnes*" (Lee et al., 2020). Bacteria commonly present on the skin are also seen.

Portillo et al. state that *Propionibacterium acnes* "has been recognized as the cause of various types of implant-associated infections, including breast implants, neurosurgical shunts, cardiovascular devices, ocular implants, internal fracture fixation devices, spinal hardware, and prosthetic joints" (Portillo et al., 2013).

Metzinger et al. examined a total of 200 patients and found that "of patients with a presentation of BII, 96% reported improved or complete resolution of their systemic symptoms after implant removal and total capsulectomy. A positive microbial culture was found in 68.5% of patients, and all culture-positive patients reported improvement post-treatment. The most common organisms found were *Propionibacterium acnes* (49.6%)" (Metzinger et al., 2022).

Notes:

Have any of your clients tested their implants after explant and found biofilm?

Mast Cells

Mast cells are part of the immune system and protect the body against a host of pathogens. Mast cells release a multitude of pro-inflammatory mediators, and one of the most important amines in mast cell granules is histamine. Gilfillan et al. state that "a wide array of bacterial products, viral products, parasite products, toxins, Toll-Like Receptor (TLR) agonists, and host defense products also induce activation of mast cells" (Gilfillan et al., 2011). Clients with mast cell issues may also be triggered by anxiety, stress, and pain.

Mast cells may also play a part in the symptoms of BII. Afrin et al. found that "some patients present with symptoms suggestive of a diagnosis of mast cell activation syndrome" (Cohen Tervaert et al., 2022). Mast cell activation syndrome (MCAS) "is a recently recognized clinical entity increasingly appreciated to be the correct root diagnosis (i.e., implying response to corresponding therapy) for a large number of patients previously found to have a large assortment of seemingly idiopathic chronic multisystem issues of general themes of inflammation ± allergic-type issues ± dystrophisms" (Afrin et al., 2020).

Miller et al. found "close correspondence" between symptom patterns for MCAS and scores on the 50-question instrument called the Quick Environmental Exposure and Sensitivity Inventory (QEESI) (Miller et al., 2021).

Notes:

Were there any interesting questions on the Qeesi that caught your attention? Why?

BII Symptoms are Similar to Those of ME/CFS and Fibromyalgia

Cohen Tervaert et al. state that "patients with BII/ASIA and fatigue often fulfill the criteria for CFS/ME, whereas patients with joint and muscle complaints fulfill the criteria for fibromyalgia and/or undifferentiated connective tissue disease" (Cohen Tervaert et al., 2022). This condition is also known as ME/CFS, which stands for Myalgic encephalomyelitis/chronic fatigue syndrome.

Cohen Tervaert et al. explain that "most patients (up to 90%) of patients with BII fulfill the classification criteria for CFS/ME. Like other patients with CFS/ME, these patients also develop symptoms of cognitive impairment resulting in debilitating symptoms such as memory deficits ('Alzheimer-light'), absent-mindedness, word-finding difficulties, and poor attention span. Most of all, these patients may also develop symptoms, which are indistinguishable from fibromyalgia, as up to 90% of these patients fulfill the 2016 classification criteria for fibromyalgia." The researchers also noted that "two-third of the patients report subjective fever-like 'pyrexia' and night sweats" (Cohen Tervaert et al., 2022).

Knowing this terminology and the symptoms of different conditions will allow massage therapists to better understand the possible origins of symptoms the client mentions on the health history form.

Notes:

Have you helped clients with ME/CFS? What treatments helped them?

Why are people getting breast implant revision surgery?

Over 131,000 people had their implants removed and replaced in 2022, and over 65,000 had their implants removed in 2022 (Aesthetic Plastic Surgery National Databank, 2023). It's important to remember that though we have learned a lot about research about symptoms of BII, all implants need to be replaced sooner or later, and most people have revision surgery because of capsular contracture. This issue of capsular contracture may be even more prevalent in our mastectomy reconstruction clients.

Let's look at the statistics from the Dutch Breast Implant Registry (DBIR). Lieffering et al. from the Netherlands wanted to know "how often do women have their silicone breast implants explanted or replaced because of breast implant illness (BII) compared with local postoperative complications?" They found that "among women who had silicone breast implants for cosmetic purposes, BII was registered as an indication for revision in 4.2% of revisions in a legacy cohort and 4.7% of revisions in a prospective cohort. Among women who had silicone breast implants for reconstructive reasons, BII was registered as the revision indication in 2.7% of revisions in a legacy cohort and 0.7% of revisions in a prospective cohort." These statistics are compared to breast revision surgery due to "capsular contracture (4775 cosmetic revisions [37.1%] and 1115 reconstruction revisions [37.9%]), followed by implant rupture in the cosmetic group (2893 revisions [22.5%]) and breast pain in the reconstructive group (714 revisions [24.2%])" (Lieffering et al., 2022).

Bottom Line:

- There are many reasons a client may choose to have breast implants removed or replaced. Capsular contracture is one of the most common complications.

Other complications include:

- Breast implant-associated anaplastic large cell lymphoma (BIA-ALCL), a type of non-Hodgkin's lymphoma,
- Very rarely, squamous cell carcinoma (SCC) can also grow in the scar tissue (capsule) that forms around breast implants,
- The FDA reports that "symptoms such as fatigue, memory loss, rash, "brain fog," and joint pain may be associated with breast implants, and some patients and clinicians may use the term "breast implant illness" to describe these symptoms or use these terms when reporting them to the FDA,
- There are several different names for the constellation of symptoms, including ASIA, BII, SSBI, and Siliconosis / Silicone Incompatibility Syndrome (SIS),
- Autoimmune/inflammatory syndrome induced by adjuvants (ASIA) is a term used more commonly outside the USA to refer to the symptoms of BII,
- BII may be caused by silicone-induced immune activation, autoimmune syndrome, biofilm and silicone toxicity,
- Heavy metals present in the breast implant may cause symptoms,
- Silicone-associated lymphadenopathy occurs following the migration of silicone particles to regional lymph nodes,

- Inflammatory response associated with the implant capsule may be more common in silicone versus saline and textured versus smooth implants,
- Biofilms may also play a role in symptoms that clients with breast implants experience,
- Clients may present with symptoms suggestive of a diagnosis of mast cell activation syndrome and/or
- Clients with BII/ASIA and fatigue often fulfill the criteria for CFS/ME and fibromyalgia.

Notes:

What does capsular contracture feel like? Dr. Youn reposted a video where levels of capsular contracture were described as feeling like a bed pillow, a decorative throw pillow, a kid's foam football, and a cue ball. https://fb.watch/qTsNBLIrDS/

Have you felt capsular contracture? What did it remind you of?

Notes:

What are the different types of implant removal surgeries?

Guimier et al. state that "capsulectomy (involving full removal of the capsule surrounding the implant) and capsulotomy (where the capsule is released and/or partly removed to create more space for the implant) are the most common surgical procedures used to treat capsular contracture" (Guimier et al., 2022). A capsulotomy is sometimes called a partial capsulectomy.

BreastCancer.org states, "During a total capsulectomy, the plastic surgeon usually removes the breast implant first and then removes the capsule in pieces. Sometimes, it's necessary for the surgeon to peel pieces of the capsule from the chest wall and surrounding tissues." The term En bloc capsulectomy describes a more involved procedure because "during an en bloc capsulectomy, the plastic surgeon makes an incision under the breast and removes the breast implant and the capsule in one piece" (Conner, 2023).

Why do some patients insist on en bloc capsulectomy? Lampert et al. state that "explant patients, especially those who are concerned for BII, often request an intact capsulectomy or an en bloc procedure regardless of the evidence-based medicine presented and awareness of increased operative time and potential risk. Concerns for occult rupture and retained silicone, persistent palpable calcified capsule, fear of BIA-ALCL, and the recent FDA safety updates on rare cases of capsular squamous cell carcinoma all may add fuel to the fire regarding patient anxiety during explant consultations" (Lampert et al., 2023).

Notes:

What is the difference between Total Capsulectomy vs Capsulectomy vs Capsulotomy?

What was interesting about the Breast Implant Removal (Explant Surgery) video?

What are Some Complications of Just Removing Breast Implants Without any Other Procedure?

Lampert et al. share that "breast implant removal, or explant, often leaves the breast with a deflated area of central hollowing, significant subsequent breast and skin laxity, loss of projection, loss of conical shape, and proportional excess in the lateral breast. Breast implant explantation alone places the patient at significant risk for resultant breast skin excess with rippling and nipple inversion as the pocket collapses down to the chest wall. Total capsulectomy with explantation likely increases the risk of these deformities, as more soft tissue is inevitably removed with the implant" (Lampert et al., 2023).

Notes:

What did you notice about the before and three month after photos of "en bloc capsulectomy?"

As a massage therapist, it is important to know what the client is talking about when they share their breast implant revision journey/explant journey, as well as what information and opinions surgeons have on the research surrounding breast implant surgery. These next two pieces of information will give you a peek into the surgeons' perspective.

It is important to know what information surgeons are receiving about the capsulectomy and en bloc procedures for patients with BII. Read this Joint Safety Statement of the International Society of Aesthetic Plastic Surgery (ISAPS), The Aesthetic Society, and The Aesthetic Surgery Education and Research Foundation (ASERF):

Patient Safety Advisory - Breast Implant Removal and Capsulectomy - https://www.theaestheticsociety.org/medical-professionals/patient-safety/patient-safety-advisory-breast-implant-removal-and-capsulectomy

Social media groups often refer to total intact capsulectomy as an 'en bloc capsulectomy' (Lampert et al., 2023). I'd like to caution you about using the term "en bloc capsulectomy" in conversations with plastic surgeons. Jacob Gerzenshtein, M.D. from the University of Central Florida College of Medicine, wrote a letter published in the Plastic and Reconstructive Surgery Journal in 2020 titled 'The Dishonesty of Referring to Total Intact Capsulectomy as "En Bloc" Resection or Capsulectomy.' He reminded surgeons that en bloc capsulectomy literally means collecting a "normal tissue margin around the capsule," which he stated would be "maiming, and that would be malpractice" (Gerzenshtein, 2020). The term en bloc capsulectomy is widely used on social media and by some surgeons to refer to just removing the entire capsule, not the capsule as well as a margin of surrounding 'normal tissue' as is done with cancer surgery. It's valuable to understand what clients mean and expect when they speak about 'en bloc' and what the term means from a medical standpoint.

Let's look at operations that remove the breast implant and also try to give the client a more pleasing cosmetic result.

If you help clients after mastectomy, you may be familiar with the deep inferior epigastric perforator (DIEP) operation. Microsurgeons can perform a DIEP flap procedure for cosmetic breast augmentation as well. In this version of the surgery, Martinez & Boutros report that "no fascia or muscle tissue was taken during flap dissection" and the surgery takes place in an outpatient setting (Martinez & Boutros, 2023).

Explant and Breast Lift Surgery/Mastopexy

Surgeons are developing procedures for achieving a better cosmetic result after capsulectomy. Let's look at one of these operations. Lampert et al. states that the Mammary Imbrication Lift and Fixation Technique is a method for "subsequent breast shaping in females electing to have their implants removed without replacement" which "allows total intact capsulectomy, preserves breast tissue and blood supply to the nipple" (Lampert et al., 2023).

According to Rand, in an auto augmentation breast lift, "the surgeon makes a T or anchor-shaped incision on the lower part of the breast as these types of incisions produce the best results long term. After the excess skin's outer layer (epidermis) is removed and tissue is adjusted, the excess breast skin and tissue that is normally discarded from the breast during a breast lift is carefully tucked back into the breast. From there the tissue is rearranged and sutured to produce a more youthful-looking shape and appearance in the breasts" (Rand, 2019).

Notes:

Fat Grafting to the Breast

Davis et al. state that liposuction and fat grafting "may also be used to provide added volume after explant surgery or to provide improvements in breast contour alongside mastopexy techniques" (Davis et al., 2020).

Where is liposuction performed? Van Boerum et al. state that "liposuction is most commonly performed in the trunk for improved contour, though it can also be performed for excess adipose tissue of the arms and legs" and "common donor sites include the abdomen, flanks, and thighs" (Van Boerum et al., 2019).

What are some complications of liposuction? Van Boerum et al. share that "one of the most common risks of liposuction is contour deformity, or rippling." This rippling is different from rippling caused by breast implants. It's also important to know that "fat grafting will typically result in 50–60% permanent take of the graft, and can be performed a number of times for optimal results" (Van Boerum et al., 2019).

Where is the grafted fat placed? Davis et al. share that "application of grafted fat to the breast may be performed directly into the pectoralis muscle or into the breast parenchyma to enhance overall breast volume and projection or more superficially to address specific contour deformities and influence local breast shape." Specific areas are targeted according to the client's needs. For instance, "cleavage appearance can be improved through fat grafting to the medial chest, which decreases the intermammary distance. In the setting of tuberous breast deformity, fat grafting can also be used unilaterally in cases of significant breast asymmetry to add volume to the underdeveloped breast" (Davis et al., 2020).

Davis et al. share that "postoperatively, it is crucial to minimize sheer forces on the breasts to allow for inosculation and revascularization of the grafted adipocytes" (Davis et al., 2020). I do not perform massage over the area of the fat graft for several weeks after the surgery. In these cases, MLD on the liposuctioned donor areas of the body (usually abdomen, flanks, back, and inner thigh are options) is indicated.

Notes:

What do you notice about the before and after photos of fat transfer to the breast?

What has your experience been with liposuction and fat transfer?

Bottom Line:

- Capsulectomy and capsulotomy are the most common surgical procedures used to treat capsular contracture.
- During a total capsulectomy, the plastic surgeon usually removes the breast implant first and then removes the capsule in pieces.
- Sometimes, it's necessary for the surgeon to peel pieces of the capsule from the chest wall and surrounding tissues.
- Social media groups often refer to total intact capsulectomy as an 'en bloc capsulectomy.'
- During a total intact or 'en bloc' capsulectomy, the plastic surgeon makes an incision under the breast and removes the breast implant and the capsule in one piece.
- Explant surgery often leaves the breast with a deflated area of central hollowing, significant subsequent breast and skin laxity, loss of projection, loss of conical shape, and proportional excess in the lateral breast.
- Explantation alone may result in breast skin excess with rippling and nipple inversion as the pocket collapses down to the chest wall.
- Some surgeons will combine explant with other procedures like flap surgery, breast lift, or fat transfer operations to give the client a more pleasing cosmetic result.

Notes:

Notes:

Let's test our memory. Describe in a sentence or two, each of the different types of breast implant surgery.

Submuscular placement

Subglandular placement

Dual plane placement

How can massage help after explant?

Acquired Macromastia and Pain with Large Breast Implants

Dr. Lukasz Swistun, a San Diego-based surgeon whose patients I see for postoperative massage, has added an interesting term to my vocabulary - acquired macromastia. This is the term he uses to describe back and neck pain that is not BII related but is like symptoms experienced by patients with an excess of breast tissue. He finds that his patients who remove their breast implants have a reduction in back and neck pain. I have also seen this in patients after a breast reduction and lift as well as after explant surgery.

Jud et al. found that "breast hypertrophy or macromastia in patients is often accompanied by several somatic problems such as chronic pain in the chest, shoulders, back, and neck, degenerative changes in the spine, and headaches. Neurological problems such as dysesthesia and carpal tunnel syndrome have been reported in the literature. Due to the skin contact between the breast and the abdomen/thorax, it is easy for irritations of the skin, eczema, and intertrigo to develop. Shortness of breath has even been reported" (Jud et al., 2020). Intertrigo is a word describing inflammation of the skin that has long-term exposure to heat and moisture, like skin at the inframammary fold.

Lonie et al. conducted a systematic review of research on reduction mammoplasty patients and found that "motivation for surgery is commonly for resolution of physical symptoms caused by the heaviness and size of breasts such as back, neck and shoulder pain, intertrigo and shoulder grooving by bra straps" and "a significant improvement in lung function tests with a positive correlation between amount of breast tissue resected and improvement in expiratory capacity" (Lonie et al., 2019).

Clients who receive breast reductions "have a sharp improvement in quality of life in the immediate post-operative period when experiencing the immediate relief of physical loss of breast weight. Patients continue to show satisfaction in the following months as they benefit both physically and psychologically from the surgery once the healing process is completed" (Lonie et al., 2019).

Breast Lift/Reduction Surgery

Coady-Fariborzian & Anstead state that "patients who experience symptomatic macromastia will report a history of neck and shoulder pain, shoulder grooving from bra straps, inframammary intertrigo, difficulty finding clothes that fit, and discomfort participating in sports" (Coady-Fariborzian & Anstead, 2021).

There are two common scar patterns in breast reduction surgery, "either vertical (periareolar plus a vertical scar from the areola to the inframammary fold) or traditional Wise pattern (also known as anchor pattern: periareolar scar, vertical scar to inframammary fold, plus a horizontal scar along the inframammary fold)."

Potential complications of breast reduction surgery can include "asymmetry, changes in nipple sensation, unattractive scars, diminished ability to breastfeed, and wound complications." Nicotine cessation is important because "smoking is a known risk factor for local wound complications in breast reduction surgery" (Coady-Fariborzian & Anstead, 2021).

Notes:

What has your experience been helping clients with macromastia and breast reduction surgery?

We have looked at the various reasons why our clients chose a certain surgery and what symptoms they may have on their health history forms as a result of their breast implants. Let's look at how we can help them recover from their surgery with massage.

Tissue Affected by Breast Implant Illness

We may feel enlarged lymph nodes, calcification, or granulomas in the tissue. The clients may also have breast pain. Cohen Tervaert et al. find that clients with breast implant illness may "describe unpleasant tingling sensations or burning pain suggestive of (atypical) small fiber neuropathy Also, unusual sensations such as 'pins-and-needles' and numbness occurs. ... Some patients have tender subcutaneous nodules in their arms, legs, abdominal wall and/or elsewhere in the body. Histologically, these nodules consists of granulomatous inflammation (i.e. migratory silicone granulomas)" (Cohen Tervaert et al., 2022).

Notes:

What has your experience been with tissue affected by breast implant illness?

Notes:

Take a look at the protocols shown in the online class.

List and describe the elements of the protocol. Why is each section important to the massage? How does each section help the client after breast implant surgery?

Notes:

Let's recap what we have learned in class. Define each of these terms in a sentence or two. What would you say to a client that asked about each condition?

Animation deformity

Bottoming out

Double bubble

Calcium deposit

Capsular contracture

Extrusion

Hematoma

Mondors

Rippling

Rupture

Seroma

Slide-down deformity

Symmastia

How might Manual Lymphatic Drainage help?

According to the Cleveland Clinic website, "lymphatic drainage massage, also known as manual lymphatic drainage, relieves swelling that happens when medical treatment or illness blocks your lymphatic system. Lymphatic drainage massage involves gently manipulating specific areas of your body to help lymph move to an area with working lymph vessels" (Lymphatic Drainage Massage, 2021).

Marxen et al. state that "some studies have incorporated MLD in their postoperative protocol for patients undergoing breast augmentation. Additionally, multiple surgeons performing mastopexy have incorporated MLD into their postoperative protocols. There are few studies evaluating the use of MLD in reduction mammaplasty, but some studies have shown altered lymphatic drainage following breast procedures, including breast reduction, suggesting a potential benefit for the incorporation of MLD into postoperative management" (Marxen et al., 2023).

MLD for Removing Waste and Reducing Stress Levels

MLD may help remove waste from tissues, reduce edema, and increase parasympathetic tone. Vairo et al. found that "manual lymphatic drainage techniques (MLDTs) are unique manual therapy interventions that may be incorporated by medical practitioners as well as allied health clinicians into rehabilitation paradigms for the treatment of somatic dysfunctions and pathologies. The theoretical bases for using such modes of manual therapy are founded on the following concepts: 1) stimulating the lymphatic system via an increase in lymph circulation, 2) expediting the removal of biochemical wastes from body tissues, 3) enhancing body fluid dynamics, thereby facilitating edema reduction, and 4) decreasing sympathetic nervous system responses while increasing parasympathetic nervous tone yielding a non-stressed body-framework state" (Vairo et al., 2009).

MLD for Balancing Hormone Levels

Antoniak et al. state that "MLD therapy reduces inflammation by lowering the release of inflammatory factors, such as prostaglandins, bradykinin and histamine. It also decreases the production of inflammatory cells, such as neutrophils, macrophages, and lymphocytes" (Antoniak et al., 2022).

A very small study by Antoniak et al. found "improvement of the concentration C-peptide, lipid profile, a reduction in the inflammation, and improved quality of life" in a patient with a BMI of 27 after a total of 10 manual lymphatic drainage (MLD) therapy sessions given three times a week for 30 minutes including "the abdominal cavity, groin area and the neck area" (Antoniak et al., 2022).

MLD for Autoimmune Issues

Sevick-Muraca et al. state that "in addition to their well-known importance in cancer and infection, the lymphatics play vital roles in the pathophysiology of many chronic conditions including rheumatoid arthritis and other autoimmune disorders, neurodegenerative diseases and chronic venous disease" (Sevick-Muraca et al., 2023).

We learned earlier that the most frequent autoimmune disease related to ASIA syndrome was UCTD. Antunes et al. say that "the term 'undifferentiated connective tissue disease' (UCTD) is generally used to describe clinical entities characterised by serological evidence of autoimmunity and by the occurrence of clinical symptoms often seen in association with systemic autoimmune diseases (SADs), yet not fulfilling criteria for a specific SAD." Indeed, the researchers state that "the use of the term UCTD to describe an early phase of a major rheumatic disease and patient who temporarily lack sufficient features to meet other classification criteria was first proposed by LeRoy *et al* in 1980" (Antunes et al., 2018).

Many clients with BII have autoimmune issues. Schwartz et al. state that "lymphatic dysfunction may contribute to the pathophysiology of rheumatic autoimmune diseases" and that "lymphatic massage techniques could be used to improve lymphatic function to help reduce tissue inflammation in autoimmune diseases" (Schwartz et al., 2019).

Why might MLD be effective for autoimmune diseases? Let's look at rheumatoid arthritis (RA). Sevick-Muraca et al. state that "preliminary clinical imaging studies of RA flare have also demonstrated altered lymphatic function, as imaged by lymphoscintigraphy and by NIRF-LI/ICG lymphography. Impaired drainage of ICG-laden lymph from the hands with dermal backflow in the wrists and forearm suggests that draining lymphatics represent a viable target for immunotherapies to quell immune responses. Indeed, lymphatic-directed treatments, including LVA and manual lymphatic drainage, represent emerging treatments for autoimmune disorders" (Sevick-Muraca et al., 2023). Lymphatic venous anastomosis (LVA) is a microsurgical treatment for lymphedema.

MLD for Breast Edema

If the client does not have a recent fat transfer to the breast, they may come to us asking for MLD on their breasts.

Let's review the lymphatic system in that area. Elahi et al. state that "there are three drainage routes of the mammary gland: the axillary ganglia, which represents the main drainage route according to Poirier, the internal mammary chain, and the supraclavicular region. Drainage blockage may result in retrograde flow to the liver" (Elahi et al., 2022).

Let's look at the lymph nodes of the breast. According to StatPearls 'Breast Lymphatics,' "75% of breast tissue drainage is into axillary lymph nodes" (Rinaldi et al. 2023).

The article "New classifications of axillary lymph nodes and their anatomical-clinical correlations in breast surgery" states that:

- Axillary lymph nodes are divided into three levels:
- I level lymph nodes are located lateral to the lateral margin of the minor pectoralis muscle.
- II level lymph nodes are located between the medial and lateral margin of the minor pectoralis muscle and the interpectoral lymph nodes.
- III level lymph nodes are located medial to the medial margin of the minor pectoralis muscle.

(Cirocchi et al., 2021).

Notes:

What has your experience been with using MLD after breast surgery? Have your clients experienced any of these effects?

MLD and Effleurage Strokes

We know that stationary circles are widely used to help interstitial fluid enter the lymphatic system. I also use effleurage strokes in my massage sessions.

Foldi & Foldi state that "Vodder style MLD consists of four techniques to stretch the skin and affect the epifascial lymph vessels. The four techniques are stationary circle, rotary, pump and scoop" (Foldi & Foldi, 2012).

In the article 'Manual lymphatic drainage: exploring the history and evidence base,' Williams shares that the Casley-Smith method "uses a slow and gentle 'effleurage,' with specific movements using the side of the hand, over the 'watershed' areas between lymphotomes (skin lymph territories)" (Williams, 2010).

Is effleurage also helping with lymphatic drainage? De Vrieze et al. found that "transport of lymph through the lymph collectors and dermal rerouting is better stimulated when the therapist glides with the hand over the skin at a relatively higher pressure than when a pumping technique at relatively lower pressure is performed" (De Vrieze et al., 2022).

The lymph collectors are an important part of reducing swelling. Belgrado et al. share that "insufficient lymphatic transport causes lymph stasis, leading to progressive swelling of the insufficiently drained anatomical area. Lymph transport is produced by mechanical forces, generated by contraction of the smooth muscle cells that are located in the collecting lymphatic wall. This contraction induces intraluminal pressure to create lymphatic pumping" (Belgrado et al., 2016).

MLD - a Surgeon's Perspective

Surgeons treating breast cancer have known about the efficacy of manual lymphatic drainage for decades. In an article published in 2007, Kirby et al. share a three part axillary and breast massage used during breast cancer surgery which "applies the principle of manual lymphatic drainage and is based on the physiology of lymphatic flow described originally by Winiwarter (1892) and Vodder (1982)." The surgeons use a blue dye to track the lymphatic fluid from the injection site to the lymph nodes in order to harvest the correct lymph node for biopsy. How does the dye work? "When injected subdermally in any area of the breast it binds to proteins and is absorbed by the lymphatics and highlights the lymphatic drainage and the sentinel lymph node in the axilla." Kirby et al. explain that "three stage lymphatic massage works containing the blue dye can be emptied easily" (Kirby et al., 2007).

Let's look at the massage techniques that surgeons use:

- In the first stage, the axilla was massaged to empty axillary lymph nodes. The lymph node massage was performed with the tips of two or three fingers. These were placed over the nodes, and pressure was applied like a gentle "scoop" in the direction of further flow from them. The fingers did not move over the skin; rather, they applied pressure during the "scoop" and released it.
- In the second stage, a retrograde massage was undertaken from the axilla towards the injection site. This was performed using the palm of the hand and fingers and light stroking movements over the skin.
- The final step was to massage from the injected area towards the axilla (Antegrade massage) to drain the blue dye into lymphatics and axillary lymph nodes.

Kirby et al. state that "the three stage massage takes about one minute to complete. It uses light-pressured strokes in a specific direction to stimulate the lymph vessels just below the surface of the skin without increasing blood circulation or reaching the depth of muscle tissue. It was thought necessary to allow about seven minutes before making the axillary incision to provide the blue dye enough time to reach the axillary glands" (Kirby et al., 2007).

What Else May Be Helpful for Clients?

What should we consider when adding other massage techniques to MLD in a massage session after breast implant removal? We can provide a customized massage that addresses the client at their current level of healing by choosing our massage strokes and modifying our massage strokes and the session itself.

First, let's look at the massage strokes we might use. I commonly use Swedish massage strokes of effleurage, petrissage, friction, and vibration. We can also use passive and active joint movement in the proliferative and maturation stages of wound healing.

When comparing a massage session after surgery to a typical relaxation massage session, I can modify several aspects of the massage itself and the session protocol to make the experience safer for a client recovering from surgery. Modifications include:

- Not working on the area of the body that received a fat transfer until cleared by their surgeon (typically 1-3 months after surgery),
- Working at a lighter pressure and shallower depth on the tissue,

- Increasing or reducing the broadness of my contact. Am I using just my fingertips or all of my fingers and the entire palm of my hand for the massage stroke? For example, using fingertips can be less invasive if pressure is light or more invasive if deeper pressure is used with a smaller focal point of massage,
- Matching the direction of my massage strokes with the direction of lymphatic flow versus strokes going in several different directions,
- Decreasing the drag on tissues,
- Decreasing the speed of the massage strokes,
- Limiting client movement during the massage to diaphragmatic breathing,
- Keep a rhythm in massage strokes, as well as slow the rhythm down. I find that meditative music helps me to keep a slower pace,
- Modifying the overall protocol of the session by ensuring I have enough time for each aspect and not rushing through sections of the massage, and
- Moving slower around the client and using eye contact and a soft, soothing voice.

I consider how both the client's tissues and their nervous system would respond to each massage modification. Some clients who had their breast implants removed because of breast implant illness may also have lingering autoimmune-related symptoms and may not heal as fast as clients with other elective surgeries. As the client's healing proceeds from the inflammatory stage to the proliferation and maturation stage, I can change or reduce each of these modifications. For instance, a client in the maturation stage can tolerate:

- Deeper pressure and depth on the tissue,
- A more focal pressure with fingers and thumbs and a deeper compression or stroke using the whole hand,
- Giving massage strokes in all directions during the massage session,
- Strokes that place drag on tissues,
- Increasing the speed of the massage strokes,
- Incorporating client-led or passive joint movement at the neck and shoulder joints,
- Faster rhythm in massage strokes and/or
- Upbeat conversation and cracking jokes.

The conversation with the plastic surgeon will often just cover the basics of the massage protocol. A fixed protocol manages the following:

- Location of massage intervention on the body (where are we massaging and where are we not massaging?).
- Frequency of massage sessions (how many sessions per week?).
- Duration of each massage session (how long is each session?) and
- Massage techniques that are off-limits (no deep tissue, no tapotement, no hydrotherapy).

Notes:

Notes:

Notes:

What did you find interesting about the video and photo of 'dents' after explant?

Wrinkles and dents after breast implant removal

What are Those Dents and Wrinkles after Capsulectomy?

What causes indentations and adhesions in breast tissue after breast implant removal? Let's see what different surgeons have to say.

On his website, Dr. Tim Sayed states that "once implants are removed, the volume of the breasts reduces significantly. This can cause several aesthetic implications:

- Breasts may appear deflated with a "sagging" appearance,
- Skin is loose and prone to extensive wrinkling,
- Nipples and areolas point downwards and/or
- Indentations and adherence to the muscle or rib cage may become evident."

Sayed states that "these issues tend to be greatest in patients with larger (more than 400cc) implants and/or smaller (less than B cup) natural breast tissue" (How do breasts look after explant surgery, n.d.).

In a Q&A section on the ASPS website, someone asked "what causes adhesions after enbloc-total capsulectemy implant removal if all scar tissue is supposed to be removed?"

Dr. Debra Johnson states that "removal of the breast implants and capsules leaves an empty space. That space has to heal back together, and that healing occurs by scar formation. Some scars tighten and can pull at the tissue, creating indentations or skin folds" (Adhesions after breast implant removal, 2019).

Johnson asks the questioner to "think of the woman who had a C-section. The scar in the lower abdomen sticks to the abdominal wall and this can create a 'shelf' where the tummy skin folds on itself. The bigger the baby, the more stretched the skin gets, and the larger the fold can be. With implants, the same situation occurs: the breast skin was enlarged by the implant. When the implants are removed there is more skin than is needed, and the scarring can cause folds or wrinkles to appear" (Adhesions after breast implant removal, 2019).

Johnson advises that surgical "remedies might include a breast lift or fat transfer. Consult with your plastic surgeon regarding options. But be sure to wait at least 6 months after the implant removal, and during that time massage the breasts to try and stretch out any adhesions" (Adhesions after breast implant removal, 2019).

In the same Q&A, Dr. Nelson Castillo states that "any time the body is forced to heal from a surgery it does so through a "scar response." Although the scar tissue around the implants were removed, your body will produce more as it attempts to heal from the procedure itself. Adhesions that are visible do not occur in all patients, so the decision to pursue a mastopexy would depend on the expectation of loose skin development after enblock capsulectomy" (Adhesions after breast implant removal, 2019).

Working with adhesions or dents after breast implant removal is working with scar tissue within the breast.

Notes:

Massage for Pain Reduction and Balancing Hormone Levels

I use Swedish massage strokes on the shoulders, neck, and upper back of clients to reduce pain and soreness from having heavy breast implants before surgery as well as sleeping in an unusual position after surgery. This part of the massage session is usually well tolerated, and clients are grateful to have their neck and back pain addressed safely at a time when getting a 'regular massage' is off-limits.

Swedish massage can also affect hormone levels. Rapaport et al. studied the effects of Swedish massage techniques, including "effleurage, petrissage, kneading, tapotement, and thumb friction," and found that when compared to a control condition, a 45-minute session of Swedish massage on a healthy client:

- Reduced whole-blood mitogen-stimulated cytokine production,
- Decreased mitogen-stimulated proinflammatory, TH-1 mediated, and TH-2 mediated cytokine levels,
- Decreased levels of arginine-vasopressin (AVP) and
- Increased the number of circulating lymphocytes, CD 25+ lymphocytes, CD 56+ lymphocytes, CD4 + lymphocytes, and CD8+ lymphocytes.

(Rapaport et al., 2010).

Why is this beneficial? Zhang & An state that "there is significant evidence showing that certain cytokines/chemokines are involved in not only the initiation but also the persistence of pathologic pain by directly activating nociceptive sensory neurons. Certain inflammatory cytokines are also involved in nerve-injury/inflammation-induced central sensitization and are related to the development of contralateral hyperalgesia/ allodynia" (Zhang & An, 2007). Additionally, arginine vasopressin (AVP) regulates water retention, and lymphocytes / white blood cells are part of our body's immune system.

Scar Massage of the Surgery Incisions

Scar massage techniques for surgical incision can usually begin 4-6 weeks after surgery. What is the purpose of scar massage? Lubczyńska et al. state that "manual scar tissue therapy uses techniques such as massage, skin rolling, cupping, myofascial release ... and instrument-assisted soft tissue mobilization to help the fiber in scar tissue and fascia to become more aligned. These techniques also reduce tension within the scar and improve blood flow to the area, which supports the healing process. The aim of the therapy is to introduce motion and nutrition to the affected tissue, which will affect the alignment of the collagen fibers" (Lubczyńska et al., 2023).

According to Lubczyńska et al., the goals of scar massage are "reducing pain and functional limitations, improving pliability, reducing hyperpigmentation, pruritus, fascial adhesions, to reduce scar thickness and smooth surface area" (Lubczyńska et al., 2023).

Why do scars need massage? Lubczyńska et al. share that "pathologic scar formation manifests itself by low tensile strength, pigment alterations, increased tension texture, and sensation irregularities. Abnormal scars arising as a result of disorders in the process of fibrosis raised above the surface of the skin, beyond the original area of damage. Often abnormal scars are accompanied by pain, itching, and contractures" (Lubczyńska et al., 2023).

Notes:

Sketch an image of the different incision sites on the breast - transaxillary, periareolar and inframammary.

Notes:

Sketch an image of the anchor scar incision pattern of a mastopexy

Adhesions

Let's talk about adhesions. Lubczyńska et al. state that "inevitable problems associated with postoperative scars are adhesions." They share that "an effective method used in anti-adhesions prevention is postoperative scar physiotherapy, including lymphatic drainage, scar mobilization ... or myofascial relaxation. Manual scar therapy to be effective requires applying physiological stimuli adequately to the phase of wound healing" (Lubczyńska et al., 2023).

Pulling, Stretching, and Negative Compression

Lubczyńska et al. state that "scar tissue massage is a form of rehabilitation that uses pulling and stretching to remodel scar tissue. Scar massage helps regain mobility and strength in damaged tissue." Scar massage should be tailored to the stage of wound healing because "overloading the scar tissue can lead to cellular damage and triggers a new inflammatory reaction" (Lubczyńska et al., 2023).

Sometimes, I will use a smaller, facial-sized cup to move the tissue on mature scars. Lubczyńska et al. share that "cupping is a supporting method used in scar treatment. Subatmospheric pressure suction affected by cup, promote peripheral blood circulation, and improve tissue elasticity. Cupping therapy can be used with caution only in the remodeling phase of the wound healing and in old scars treatment. The reported effect of cupping therapy includes modification of the skin's biomechanical properties and improving local anaerobic metabolism" (Lubczyńska et al., 2023).

Remember from earlier in class that adhesions in the breast tissue are also scar tissue. We can apply many of the same theories and techniques to these tissues as well.

There are many excellent in-person and online training classes in scar massage, including classes that specialize in scar massage of the breast after breast cancer surgery.

Notes:

Massage after Fat Transfer to the Breast

Many of my explant clients also have liposuction and fat transfer to breasts. Lieffering et al. state that "fat grafting was a frequently used technique in addition to explantation because of BII" (Lieffering et al., 2022).

What can help in the healing process after liposuction? Dixit & Wagh state that "some of the methods that are commonly employed to minimise post-operative oedema [swelling, or edema] are: applying an optimum compressive garment immediately after surgery... providing manual lymphatic drainage in the early post-operative period. In our experience gentle liposuctioning, an optimum compressive garment and early lymphatic drainage massage helps to accelerate the clearance of oedema" (Dixit & Wagh, 2013).

People have used MLD to heal from plastic surgery for over 25 years. In the presentation "Manual Lymphatic Drainage Therapy: An Integral Component of Postoperative Care in Plastic Surgery Patients," given at the first annual conference of the American Society of Lymphology, Dr. Casas and Dr. DePoli (1999) found that when clients recovering from surgery (liposuction of the abdomen, buttocks, hips or thighs, abdominoplasty/tummy tuck, or facelift) were treated with MLD and deep tissue massage 1–2 times per week for the first 3–6 weeks following their operation, with deep tissue massage given as subcutaneous fibrosis developed, they recovered faster. Fibrosis is the thickening or scarring of connective tissue in the body.

Marxen et al. state that "numerous studies have found that MLD in conjunction with therapeutic adjuncts can provide reductions in edema, fibrosis, as well as provided analgesia in patients undergoing liposuction and/or lipoabdominoplasty. These been found to extended from the abdomen to all core liposuction areas, including the upper and lower abdomen, flanks, back, and hips" (Marxen et al., 2023).

The liposuction area may feel lumpy during the healing process. Dixit & Wagh outline four reasons for lumps and bumps after liposuction:

- liposuction too close to the surface of the skin,
- fibrotic adhesions,
- loose skin, and/or
- not wearing the compression garment properly.

(Dixit & Wagh, 2013).

How Can We Tell these Reasons Apart?

Dixit and Wagh say "surface dents due to excessive superficial liposuction persist on skin retraction and in the supine position. Dents due to fibrous adhesions to underlying muscle worsen on muscle contraction and dents due to skin redundancy may improve on supine position but will definitely improve on skin retraction" (Dixit & Wagh, 2013). McNemar et al. say treatment of the inner thighs often brings less even results than the outer thigh because "the thin, delicate skin on the inner thighs is more likely to reveal any irregularities or unevenness under the skin" (McNemar et al., 2006).

Bottom Line:

- Massage on the area of the body that received a fat transfer is contraindicated until cleared by the surgeon.
- 75% of breast tissue drainage is into axillary lymph nodes.
- MLD may help remove waste from tissues, reduce edema and increase parasympathetic tone.
- MLD may stimulate the lymphatic system via an increase in lymph circulation.
- MLD may expedite the removal of biochemical wastes from body tissues.
- MLD may enhance body fluid dynamics, thereby facilitating edema reduction.
- MLD may decrease sympathetic nervous system responses while increasing parasympathetic nervous tone yielding a non-stressed body-framework state.
- MLD reduces inflammation by lowering the release of inflammatory factors, such as prostaglandins, bradykinin and histamine.
- MLD decreases the production of inflammatory cells, such as neutrophils, macrophages, and lymphocytes.
- Transport of lymph through the lymph collectors and dermal rerouting is better stimulated when the therapist glides with the hand over the skin at a relatively higher pressure.
- Swedish massage can affect hormone levels.
- Breast hypertrophy or macromastia in patients is often accompanied by several somatic problems such as chronic pain in the chest, shoulders, back, and neck, degenerative changes in the spine, and headaches.

- Removing breast implants can result in breast tissue wrinkling, indentations and adherence to the muscle or rib cage.
- Working with adhesions or dents after breast implant removal is working with scar tissue within the breast.
- Cupping is a supporting method used in scar treatment.
- Scar massage can help scar tissue and fascia to become aligned.
- Scar massage can reduce tension, pain, itching and adhesions.
- Scar massage can improve blood flow and range of motion.
- One of the most common risks of liposuction is contour deformity or rippling.
- Fat grafting to the breast using liposuction will typically result in 50–60% permanent take of the graft.
- Common liposuction fat grafting donor sites include the abdomen, flanks and thighs.
- Lumps and bumps after liposuction may be due to liposuction too close to the surface of the skin, fibrotic adhesions, loose skin and/or not wearing the compression garment properly.
- Surface dents due to excessive superficial liposuction persist on skin retraction and in the supine position.
- Dents due to fibrous adhesions to underlying muscle worsen on muscle contraction.
- Dents due to skin redundancy may improve on supine position, but will definitely improve on skin retraction.

Notes:

How can we optimize our massage therapy office to help these clients?

Massage Room Supplies:

Have facial tissues on hand.

Clients may need to blow their nose, especially clients with breast implant illness. Cohen Tervaert et al. state that "atopic symptoms, such as sneezing, a runny nose, itchy eyes, red eyes, nasal congestion and post nasal drip, are also common and are reported in 50–80% of patients. Although allergies may be preexistent, many patients report exacerbation of their symptoms that were minimal prior to implantation" (Cohen Tervaert et al., 2022).

Use caution with flowers/scents, pet hair, latex gloves, and metal.

Many clients with BII have allergies. Cohen Tervaert et al. state that "allergies that are frequently observed are pollen allergy, pet allergy, mold allergy, latex allergy, and food allergy" and "metal-allergy is documented presenting as an itchy rash after exposure to nickel-containing substances" (Cohen Tervaert et al., 2022).

Silicone cups - be aware that some women will be afraid and concerned if you attempt to use silicone cups or anything with silicone during the massage. Clients may also be hesitant to use silicone cream or scar strips on their scars.

Bathroom Access

Some BII clients may also have interstitial cystitis. According to Cohen Tervaert et al., symptoms may include "bladder pressure, bladder pain, and sometimes pelvic pain often accompanied by urinary symptoms, such as urgency or frequency" (Cohen Tervaert et al., 2022). I have a size extra-large housecoat/bathrobe in my massage room that clients can use if they have to use the bathroom during their massage session.

Positioning on the Massage Table and Cautions

Cohen Tervaert et al. have found that people with breast implant illness may have "signs of orthostatic intolerance such as dizziness, disturbed balance, irregular heartbeat, and sometimes chest pain. Tilt testing may reveal a diagnosis of POTS (Postural Orthostatic Tachycardia Syndrome)" (Cohen Tervaert et al., 2022).

POTS clients may experience dizziness getting up off the table after their massage.

Cohen Tervaert et al. have found "a mitral valve prolapse and/or joint hypermobility is found in about half of the patients" with breast implant illness (Cohen Tervaert et al., 2022). Clients may mention they are hypermobile and know their Beighton Score number. Be cautious with moving these clients' joints or applying stretches as they may have increased range of motion at their joints.

"T-Rex arms"

Clients may have movement restrictions for their arms for six weeks as the surgery heals, including only being able to lift a few pounds and strict orders to not reach or raise their arms overhead. Clients may also have to avoid lying prone if they have had a fat transfer to the breasts. Remember - many breast augmentation surgeries include surgery on the pectoralis major muscle! I usually ask them how they sleep or nap and replicate that position for the massage.

Lower Body Bolstering

If the client seems especially anxious, I may use a wedge to elevate the entire lower leg above the heart to encourage a parasympathetic nervous system response (Søndergaard, 2022).

Appointment Reminders

My massage software sends clients a reminder the day before their appointment. The 'brain fog' symptoms may make it difficult for clients to remember their appointments. One client joked (a little too seriously) that it would help if I texted her when it was time to leave the house before the appointment.

Notes:

Health History Form

What are some things to keep in mind as we look at the client's health history form?

Mast Cell and Anxiety

Clients with mast cell issues may benefit from reducing stress before and after their surgery and avoiding breakthrough pain. Nicoloro-SantaBarbara et al. state that "when mast cells are activated, they release pro-inflammatory substances which can lead to a wide variety of symptoms including anaphylaxis, fatigue, headache, angioedema, flushing, rash/hives, diarrhea, uterine cramps or bleeding, shortness of breath, blood pressure instability, acid reflux, muscle and bone pain, syncope, brain fog, and flushing" (Nicoloro-SantaBarbara et al., 2021).

What may set off mast cell activation? Nicoloro-SantaBarbara et al. say that "potential triggers of mast cell activation include heat/cold, emotional and physical stress including pain, exercise, fatigue, foods and beverages, medications, infections, and venom" (Nicoloro-SantaBarbara et al., 2021).

Autoimmune Disorders

BII clients may also have autoimmune or rheumatic disorders. The Watad study, which included over 24,000 women with silicone breast implants and over 98,000 matched controls without silicone breast implants, found that "26.4% of women with breast implants had an autoimmune/rheumatic disorder. They calculated that women with breast implants had a 45% increased risk for being diagnosed with at least one autoimmune/rheumatic disorder, compared to those without breast implants" (Cohen Tervaert et al., 2022).

Hearing Difficulty

Greenbaum et al. interviewed 160 women with silicone breast implants (SBI) and found that "hearing impairment is a frequent complaint among symptomatic women with SBIs, and tinnitus was found to be the most common complaint." Tinnitus is the "perception of sound in the absence of an external auditory stimulus." The researchers also mention that some study participants "exhibited high-frequency sensory neural hearing loss. This finding is in keeping with the results of a recent review on audiologic manifestations of autoimmune inner ear diseases" (Greenbaum et al., 2023).

Frailty

If you see frailty, be on the lookout for surgical site infections. Liu et al. found a link between higher surgical site infections and higher modified 5-item frailty index (mFI-5) score in clients undergoing breast implant augmentation surgery and is associated with overall complications. Researchers have also found that "increasing mFI-5 scores was significantly associated with postoperative complications" in "breast reconstruction, free-flap procedures and mastectomies" (Liu et al., 2023).

The modified 5-item frailty index (mFI-5) includes questions about:

- Diabetes mellitus,
- Hypertension requiring medication,
- Chronic obstructive pulmonary disease (COPD),

- Congestive heart failure and
- The ability to carry out activities of daily living (functional status).

Kim et al. performed an analysis of over 2,00 patients and found that "the 5-item modified frailty index (mFI-5) was developed to measure frailty and it has been shown to be a powerful predictor of complications after breast reconstruction, especially after autologous-based reconstruction (ABR)." The components of the MFI-5 in this study also included "a diagnosis of pneumonia within 30 days" (M. Kim et al., 2024).

Notes:

Medications

The medications portion of the client's health history form may be long, especially if the client has breast implant illness. Let's look at some of the medications we might see on the client's form and learn more about why they may have been prescribed.

If the client is unusually swollen, I always recheck their list of medications. Prescription medications can have an effect on swelling, including calcium antagonists, some steroids, NSAIDs, sex hormones, anticonvulsants (gabapentin), anti-parkinson, anti-diabetes, and biphosphates. I advise clients to discuss any concerns with their physician and pharmacist.

Antibiotics

The client's postoperative medications usually include antibiotics. Antibiotics can have an effect on digestion. Ramirez et al. state that "antibiotic use can have several negative effects on the gut microbiota, including reduced species diversity, altered metabolic activity, and the selection of antibiotic-resistant organisms, which in turn can lead to antibiotic-associated diarrhea and recurrent *Clostridioides difficile* infection"(CDI). Which drugs have the most side effects? The researchers state that "the most significant risk factor for CDI is antibiotic use, with the most commonly associated drugs being ampicillin, amoxicillin, cephalosporins, clindamycin, and fluoroquinolones" (Ramirez et al., 2020).

Probiotics

Clients may also be taking probiotics because studies have shown that "the incidence of CDI is lower in adult patients who receive probiotics in addition to antibiotic treatment than in those who received placebo" (Ramirez et al., 2020).

Gao et al. also state that "orally taking of probiotics drugs during radiotherapy, chemotherapy and surgery in patients can significantly reduce their side effects by improving the disorder of intestinal microbiota. Other works also indicated that dietary supplements (prebiotics) or prebiotics could selectively stimulate the growth and activity of internal probiotics to reduce the disorder of intestinal microbiota" (Gao et al., 2020).

Medications to Prevent Capsular Contracture of Breast Implants

Huang & Handel share that "capsular contracture (CC) is one of the most common complications of breast augmentation surgery. Leukotrienes are implicated in the inflammatory cascade and have been postulated to be involved in the formation of CC. Therefore, leukotriene antagonists Accolate and Singulair have been prescribed by plastic surgeons off-label to treat and prevent CC" (Huang & Handel, 2010). A meta-analysis of five studies involving 1710 breast prosthesis implantations by Wang et al. "demonstrated that leukotriene antagonists (montelukast and zafirlukast) have significant effects in treating and preventing capsular contracture" (Wang et al., 2020). Papaconstantinou et al. state that "the use of zafirlukast must be monitored carefully because normal doses have been reported to cause liver failure manifesting as anorexia, right upper quadrant pain, pruritus, or jaundice" (Papaconstantinou et al., 2020).

Nightmares and suicidal ideation may be side effects of Montelukast. Have clients speak to their surgeon immediately if they are experiencing this suicidal ideation (Watson et al., 2022).

Other medications that may be used to treat capsular contracture include:

- Diclofenac is a patch containing "nonsteroidal anti-inflammatory drug (NSAID)." Le Louarn et al. found that "approximately 3 weeks of treatment, a high frequency of change from capsular contracture Baker 2 or 3 to Baker 1 occurs, provided the application was started no later than 3 months after the onset of capsular contracture" (Le Louarn et al., 2008).
- Pirfenidone is an "antifibrotic, cytokine, and extracellular matrix (ECM) degradation modulator" and Veras-Castillo et al. state that it has "minor side effects like photosensitivity, nausea, vomiting, and gastric discomfort resolved after 2 to 3 months of intake" (Veras-Castillo et al., 2013).
- Salinomycin is an "antibacterial and anticoccidial drug" (Qi et al., 2022). It may have benefits for capsular contracture after radiation. Hansen et al. found that "ionizing radiation-induced Thy1 over-expression may contribute to increased capsular contracture severity, and fibroblast scar production can be ameliorated through targeting Thy1 expression. Importantly, our new results show promise for the anti-scarring ability of salinomycin in radiation-induced capsular contracture." They found that "radiated capsule showed higher Thy1 mRNA and protein levels, but *in vivo* blockade using Salinomycin resulted in reduced scar component production and a phenotypic disruption of myofibroblast transformation" (Hansen et al., 2017).

- Simvastatin is a 3-hydroxy-3-methylglutaryl-coenzyme A (HMG-CoA) reductase inhibitor and Chung et al. state it is commonly prescribed for "reducing cholesterol levels and improving serum lipid profiles. In recent years, simvastatin has also been found to have pleiotropic effects, including immunomodulatory and anti-inflammatory effects" and has been found to reduce "radiation-induced capsular fibrosis around silicone implants in rats" (Chung et al., 2016). Yin et al. state that Simvastatin has also "demonstrated significant beneficial effects in reducing breast cancer metastasis and recurrence" (Yin et al., 2020).
- Blum et al. found that "Tamoxifen treatment in the mouse silicone breast implant model decreased capsule formation through modulation of myofibroblasts, neovascularization, and collagen deposition. Tamoxifen may be useful for reducing or preventing capsule formation in clinical breast implantations" (Blum et al., 2022).
- Cook et al. found that "the combination of Trental and vitamin E can prevent severe contracture and implant losses allowing for immediate reconstruction with implant or tissue expander even if radiation is planned after mastectomy" (Cook et al., 2016).
- Triamcinolone may be injected into the capsule. Papaconstantinou et al. treated with triamcinolone "reported four major complications: one implant puncture and three major atrophies and several minor complications (mainly thinning of the skin)" (Papaconstantinou et al., 2020).

Notes:

My notes of side effects of medications:

Pain Medications

Clients may be prescribed one or several pain medications after their surgery. Let's learn how some common pain medications work and their side effects.

NSAID

Clients may be prescribed a non-steroidal anti-inflammatory drug (NSAID) or non-opioid analgesics for pain relief. They may also be directed to take an over the counter NSAID like ibuprofen or naproxen. One prescription drug is Celebrex.

Also, read the Anxiety/Depression Medications section for information on bleeding and NSAIDs.

Anticoagulants

If clients are at risk for a blood clot, they may be put on anticoagulants. This will thin their blood and make them susceptible to easy bruising. Do not give these clients deep tissue or vigorous, firm massage!

Eliquis is one medication your clients may be prescribed.

Anxiety/Depression Medications

It's important to know that clients on medication for anxiety and depression may have an increased risk of bleeding. Edinoff et al. state that "Selective Serotonin Reuptake Inhibitors (SSRI) inhibit serotonin reuptake and subsequently increase the amount of serotonin available in synapses" and "the inhibition of serotonin reuptake can affect platelet aggregation since platelets also express the serotonin transporter." SSRI medications used in the USA "include fluvoxamine, fluoxetine, sertraline, paroxetine, citalopram, escitalopram, and vilazodone" (Edinoff et al., 2022).

What are the side effects of SSRIs? The researchers state that "increased serotonin can also increase gastric acid secretion, which increases the risk for ulceration. SSRIs in combination with NSAIDs also show a significantly increased risk of upper GI bleeding." Edinoff et al. state that "another population that showed an increased bleeding risk is post-breast augmentation surgery. Hematomas typically present within a week of surgery and can be severe enough to need surgical drainage and medical treatment. The most common complication is hematomas from drugs such as platelet inhibitors, vitamin K antagonists, oral anticoagulants, estrogen, and NSAIDs. However, SSRIs are still considered a player in hematoma formation. The global incidence of post breast augmentation surgery hematomas is reported to be 1.44%, while patients who were taking SSRIs had an incidence of 4.59%" (Edinoff et al., 2022).

Granuloma Medications

Harlim et al. found that "when the granuloma cannot be removed, other modalities can be given after wound healing period," including:

- Allopurinol,
- Etanercept,
- Topical imiquimod,
- Minocycline,
- Topical treatment of pimetacrolimus,
- Oral prednisone and
- Intralesion corticosteroid injection of triamcinolone.

(Harlim et al., 2018).

Notes:

My notes of side effects of medications:

Topical Products, Binders and Supplements

Clients may be directed to use a scar cream or lotion containing arnica after surgery. Another product is called ReFORM & RePAIR with TriHex Technology (Alastin) and, according to Casas et al., is a "peri-surgical product designed for the use with invasive surgery" which "produced significant differences in ecchymosis, skin discoloration, edema, induration and ongoing resolution of fibrous banding over many weeks." Interestingly, MLD therapists found that clients who used this in a double blind trial had less need for MLD in the area the product was used (Casas et al., 2022). This product does contain Dimethicone, which is silicone based. It also contains Centella Asiatica Extract, which is also known as Gotu Kola. Ratz Lyco et al., state that "*Centella asiatica* extract is a rich source of natural bioactive substances, triterpenoid saponins, flavonoids, phenolic acids, triterpenic steroids, amino acids and sugars. Thus, many scavenging free radicals, exhibit antiinflammatory activity and affect on the *stratum corneum* hydration and epidermal barrier function" (Ratz Lyco et al., 2016).

Supplements

Clients may also be taking supplements for general wellness, to treat the symptoms of breast implant illness or to help in healing after their surgery.

Binders / Sequestering Agents

I first heard of the practice of using 'binders' when 'detoxing' from breast implant illness groups on Facebook and social media. Hope states that "sequestering agents refer to nonabsorbable materials capable of binding toxins in the gastrointestinal tract, thus reducing enterohepatic recirculation and ultimately the body burden of toxins. These agents are not absorbed into systemic circulation; therefore, side effects are typically limited to gastrointestinal symptoms." If a client is taking sequestering agents like activated carbons and chlorella at the wrong times, they can also bind "medications, vitamins, and nutrients and should be taken several hours apart from medications and vitamins and ideally on an empty stomach" (Hope, 2013).

Notes:

What have I heard from my clients or online about binders?

Other Supplements

Ashwagandha - this ayurvedic herb is used for many conditions in India. Paul et al. state that a "comparative analysis of relevant in-vitro, in-vivo, and clinical investigations indicated potent bioactivity of W. somnifera extracts and phytochemicals as anti-cancer, anti-inflammatory, apoptotic, immunomodulatory, antimicrobial, anti-diabetic, hepatoprotective, hypoglycaemic, hypolipidemic, cardio-protective" (Paul et al., 2021).

Fish oil / Omega 3 - Lombardo et al. found that "omega-3 supplementation seems to be effective in reducing the occurrence of capsular formation, mainly through inhibition of the TGF-β pathway and impairment of collagen deposit" (Lombardo et al., 2020).

Glutathione, according to Kennedy et al., is a "intracellular antioxidant, it acts as a regulator of cellular redox state protecting cells from damage caused by lipid peroxides, reactive oxygen and nitrogen species, and xenobiotics" (Kennedy et al., 2020).

Milk thistle / Silymarin - researchers state that "the active substance in milk thistle, silymarin, is a complex mixture of flavonolignans" and "laboratory studies demonstrate that silymarin stabilizes cellular membranes, stimulates detoxification pathways, stimulates regeneration of liver tissue." Research via "laboratory experiments conducted using cancer cell lines have suggested that silibinin enhances the efficacy of cisplatin and doxorubicin against ovarian and breast cancer cells" (PDQ, 2022).

N-acetyl cysteine (NAC) - according to Raghu et al., "N-acetylcysteine (NAC) is a synthetic derivative of the endogenous amino acid L-cysteine (Fig. 1), and a precursor of GSH. NAC not only modulates oxidative stress but other pathophysiologic processes implicated in disease. These include mitochondrial dysfunction, apoptosis, and inflammation, as well as indirect effects on neurotransmitters such as glutamate and dopamine." NAC also may have an effect on mitochondrial dysfunction and heavy metal neurotoxicity. (Raghu et al., 2021)

Notes:

What have I heard from my clients or online about supplements?

Autoimmune Disease Medications

Marwa & Anjum state that drug treatments for undifferentiated connective tissue disease include nonsteroidal anti-inflammatory drugs, corticosteroids, calcium channel blockers, and antimalarial drugs such as hydroxychloroquine" (Marwa & Anjum, 2023).

- "Azathioprine is typically effective for joint and extra-articular symptoms" (Marwa & Anjum, 2023).
- "Antimalarial drugs are usually used in case of a severe rash or photosensitivity. These drugs have anti-chemotactic effects on inflammatory leukocytes. They can prevent intracellular processing of the autoantigens... Hydroxychloroquine is a common example, and it can inhibit the chemotaxis of neutrophils and eosinophils, which prevent the activation of complement systems" (Marwa & Anjum, 2023).
- "Calcium channel blockers are commonly used in connective tissue diseases. They can relax the vascular smooth muscles and decrease the resistance of peripheral vessels, which helps in the management of the Raynaud phenomenon. Nifedipine and diltiazem are examples of calcium channel blockers" (Marwa & Anjum, 2023).
- "Methotrexate is considered a steroid-sparing agent. This drug decreases symptoms of inflammation associated with undifferentiated connective tissue disease" (Marwa & Anjum, 2023).
- "NSAIDs can be useful for their antipyretic, analgesic, and anti-inflammatory effects. Naproxen is a good example, and it is used for mild-to-moderate pain relief. Another choice is COX-2 selective medication such as celecoxib, which is used to minimize adverse effects seen with non-

selective NSAIDs as gastric ulcers and gastrointestinal bleeding" (Marwa & Anjum, 2023)

- "Prednisone is a common type of systemic corticosteroid and is considered an immunosuppressant agent. It is often used for autoimmune disorders since it can decrease the inflammation caused by the immune system" (Marwa & Anjum, 2023).

Notes:

Side effects of medications:

Hormone Therapy

Bekeny et al. state that "while not required, transgender patients are recommended to take exogenous hormones for at least 1 year before undergoing surgical breast augmentation; coordination with an endocrinologist or primary care doctor experienced with transgender patient care is recommended. The addition of exogenous hormones, can lead to an increase in parenchymal breast tissue, leading to a better cosmetic outcome after breast augmentation" (Bekeny et al., 2020).

What hormones will we find in the health history form? Bekeny et al. state that "the most common type of exogenous hormone involves 17-β estradiol, which is often taken orally in doses of 2 to 6 mg per day, but anti-androgens and other formulations are also commonly used. Exogenous estrogens may be stopped 2–4 weeks preceding surgery to reduce risk of thromboembolism" (Bekeny et al., 2020).

People experiencing perimenopause or menopause may also be taking sex hormones to counteract the symptoms of menopause. These hormones may be applied topically as a cream or in a patch.

Notes:

What have I heard from my clients or online about hormones?

Bottom Line:

- Many plastic surgeons recommend manual lymphatic drainage / lymphatic massage after surgery, including explant surgery.
- We can make modifications to our massage office to support these clients.
- We should be aware of side effects of mast cell issues, POTS, frailty and other medical issues.
- The medications portion of the client's health history form may be long, especially if the client has breast implant illness.
- They may be on medications to treat autoimmune disease and other issues if they have breast implant illness.
- They may also be taking medications that may be used to prevent or treat capsular contracture.
- Researchers state that drug treatments for undifferentiated connective tissue disease include nonsteroidal anti-inflammatory drugs, corticosteroids, calcium channel blockers, and antimalarial drugs such as hydroxychloroquine.
- Clients undergoing gender affirmation surgery may be taking exogenous hormones before undergoing surgical breast augmentation.
- Clients experiencing menopause and perimenopause may also be on hormone therapy.

Notes:

Conclusion

The Breast Massage after Implant and Explant Plastic Surgery class focused on evidence-based practices for using manual lymphatic drainage (MLD) and other types of massage to help clients reduce pain and swelling after surgery involving breast implants. We looked at a few different types of surgery, including:

Breast implant surgery for cosmetic reasons

Breast implant surgery for gender affirmation / top surgery

Implant-based reconstruction after mastectomy

Removal of breast implants for cosmetic and health reasons

Before taking the quiz, please be comfortable:

- Describing popular plastic surgery procedures involving breast implants,
- Discussing complications and experiences of patients after breast surgery,
- Explaining contraindications to post-surgery breast massage,
- Describing the stages of wound healing and matching the massage intervention to the client's current stage of wound healing, and
- Describing massage modalities that can reduce swelling and other side effects of surgery.

Using the protocols provided in the online class as inspiration and incorporating your own massage skills, you should be able to design a sample session for a client recovering from breast surgery based on your current knowledge and skills.

Compared to a session of relaxation massage for a healthy client, a session of massage after breast implant related surgery involves:

- Not working on the area of the body that received a fat transfer until cleared by their surgeon (typically 1-3 months after surgery),
- Working within the clients' restrictions on shoulder range of motion and elevating the client's upper or lower body if indicated,
- Obtaining additional written and verbal permission for breast massage when working on the breast,
- Observing contraindications to massage,
- Working at a lighter pressure and shallower depth on the tissue,
- Increasing or reducing the broadness of contact to avoid deep pressure,
- Matching the direction of massage strokes with the direction of lymphatic flow versus strokes going in several directions over the length of the massage session,
- Decreasing the drag on tissues,
- Decreasing the speed of the massage strokes,
- Limiting client joint movement during the massage to diaphragmatic breathing,
- Keeping a rhythm in massage strokes, as well as slowing the rhythm down,
- Modifying the overall protocol of the session by ensuring enough time for each aspect and not rushing through sections of the massage, and
- Moving slower around the client and using eye contact and a soft, soothing voice.

You should feel more comfortable and confident when speaking with clients about breast implant related plastic surgery procedures, including their side effects and how massage can benefit client recovery.

Notes:

Research

8 Signs of Wound Infection. (2016 Oct. 19). Retrieved from: https://www.woundsource.com/blog/8-signs-wound-infection

Acellular Dermal Matrix (ADM) Products Used in Implant-Based Breast Reconstruction Differ in Complication Rates: FDA Safety Communication (2021 Mar. 31) Retrieved from: https://www.fda.gov/medical-devices/safety-communications/acellular-dermal-matrix-adm-products-used-implant-based-breast-reconstruction-differ-complication

Adhesions after breast implant removal (2019). Retrieved from: https://www1.plasticsurgery.org/psconnect/askasurgeon/detail.aspx?thread=562

Aesthetic Plastic Surgery National Databank Statistics (2023). Retrieved from: https://cdn.theaestheticsociety.org/media/statistics/2022-TheAestheticSocietyStatistics.pdf

Afrin LB, Ackerley MB, Bluestein LS, Brewer JH, Brook JB, Buchanan AD, Cuni JR, Davey WP, Dempsey TT, Dorff SR, Dubravec MS, Guggenheim AG, Hindman KJ, Hoffman B, Kaufman DL, Kratzer SJ, Lee TM, Marantz MS, Maxwell AJ, McCann KK, McKee DL, Menk Otto L, Pace LA, Perkins DD, Radovsky L, Raleigh MS, Rapaport SA, Reinhold EJ, Renneker ML, Robinson WA, Roland AM, Rosenbloom ES, Rowe PC, Ruhoy IS, Saperstein DS, Schlosser DA, Schofield JR, Settle JE, Weinstock LB, Wengenroth M, Westaway M, Xi SC, Molderings GJ. Diagnosis of mast cell activation syndrome: a global „consensus-2“. Diagnosis (Berl). 2020 Apr 22;8(2):137-152. doi: 10.1515/dx-2020-0005. PMID: 32324159.

Amano M, Shimizu T. Mondor's Disease: A Review of the Literature. Intern Med. 2018 Sep 15;57(18):2607-2612. doi: 10.2169/internalmedicine.0495-17. Epub 2018 May 18. PMID: 29780120; PMCID: PMC6191595.

Antoniak K, Zorena K, Hansdorfer-Korzon R, Wojtowicz D, Koziński M. Favourable Changes in C-Peptide, C-Reactive Protein and Lipid

Profile, and Improved Quality of Life in Patients with Abnormal Body Mass Index after the Use of Manual Lymphatic Drainage: A Case Series with Three-Month Follow-Up. Medicina (Kaunas). 2022 Feb 11;58(2):273. doi: 10.3390/medicina58020273. PMID: 35208596; PMCID: PMC8878077.

Antunes M, Scirè CA, Talarico R, Alexander T, Avcin T, Belocchi C, Doria A, Franceschini F, Galetti I, Govoni M, Hachulla E, Launay D, Lepri G, Macieira C, Matucci-Cerinic M, Montecucco CM, Moraes-Fontes MF, Mouthon L, Paolino S, Ramoni V, Tani C, Tas SW, Tincani A, Van Vollenhoven R, Zen M, Fonseca J, Bombardieri S, Fonseca JE, Schneider M, Smith V, Cutolo M, Mosca M, Beretta L. Undifferentiated connective tissue disease: state of the art on clinical practice guidelines. RMD Open. 2019 Feb 26;4(Suppl 1):e000786. doi: 10.1136/rmdopen-2018-000786. PMID: 30886731; PMCID: PMC6397427.

Azis KA, Al-Chalabi MMM, Mat Johar SFN, Wan Sulaiman WA. Atypical Chest Pain in a Patient With Breast Implant. Cureus. 2023 Apr 18;15(4):e37751. doi: 10.7759/cureus.37751. PMID: 37214021; PMCID: PMC10193515.

Beer, K., Lupo, M. P., & Narurkar, V. A. (2011). *Cosmetic Bootcamp Primer Comprehensive Aesthetic Management*. Informa Healthcare.

Belgrado JP, Vandermeeren L, Vankerckhove S, Valsamis JB, Malloizel-Delaunay J, Moraine JJ, Liebens F. Near-Infrared Fluorescence Lymphatic Imaging to Reconsider Occlusion Pressure of Superficial Lymphatic Collectors in Upper Extremities of Healthy Volunteers. Lymphat Res Biol. 2016 Jun;14(2):70-7. doi: 10.1089/lrb.2015.0040. Epub 2016 May 11. PMID: 27167187; PMCID: PMC4926199.

Belgrado JP, Bonetti G, Maloizelle-Delaunay J, Stoichkova V, Tartaglia GM, Chiurazzi P, Cecchin S, Bertelli M. Lymphatic circulation in astronauts: basic knowledge, challenges and perspectives. Eur Rev Med Pharmacol Sci. 2023 Dec;27(6 Suppl):119-126. doi: 10.26355/eurrev_202312_34696. PMID: 38112952.

Bekeny JC, Zolper EG, Fan KL, Del Corral G. Breast augmentation for transfeminine patients: methods, complications, and outcomes. Gland Surg. 2020 Jun;9(3):788-796. doi: 10.21037/gs.2020.03.18. PMID: 32775269; PMCID: PMC7347817.

Blum KM, Mirhaidari GJM, Zbinden JC, Breuer CK, Barker JC. Tamoxifen reduces silicone implant capsule formation in a mouse model. FASEB Bioadv. 2022 Aug 16;4(10):638-647. doi: 10.1096/fba.2022-00036. PMID: 36238364; PMCID: PMC9536088.

Botox Injections (2023). Retrieved from: https://www.mayoclinic.org/tests-procedures/botox/about/pac-20384658

Brazin J, Malliaris S, Groh B, Mehrara B, Hidalgo D, Otterburn D, Silver RB, Spector JA. Mast cells in the periprosthetic breast capsule. Aesthetic Plast Surg. 2014 Jun;38(3):592-601. doi: 10.1007/s00266-014-0318-2. Epub 2014 May 9. PMID: 24811971.

Breast Implants (2023). Retrieved from:

https://www.fda.gov/medical-devices/implants-and-prosthetics/breast-implants

Breast Reconstruction With a Flap: What to Expect at Home (n.d.). https://myhealth.alberta.ca/health/AfterCareInformation/pages/conditions.aspx?hwid=tw12584

Bresnick SD. Management of a Common Breast Augmentation Complication: Treatment of the Double-Bubble Deformity With Fat Grafting. Ann Plast Surg. 2016 Jan;76(1):18-22. doi: 10.1097/SAP.0000000000000553. PMID: 26101976; PMCID: PMC4679341.

Briot N, Chagnon G, Burlet L, Gil H, Girard E, Payan Y. Experimental characterisation and modelling of breast Cooper's ligaments. Biomech Model Mechanobiol. 2022 Aug;21(4):1157-1168. doi: 10.1007/s10237-022-01582-5. Epub 2022 Apr 28. PMID: 35482144; PMCID: PMC9047630.

Casas, L. & DePoli, P. (1999). Manual lymphatic drainage therapy: An integral component of postoperative care in plastic surgery patients. *Proceedings of The First Annual Conference of the American Society of Lymphology.* 1999 Aug. Chicago.

Casas LA, Claytor RB, Zeidler KR, Shridharani SM, Cohen SR, Khanna JJ, Gould DJ, Yates EK, Lultschik S, Bell M, Widgerow AD. A Multicenter, Randomized, Double-Blind, Split-Body Clinical Trial Evaluating the Efficacy and Outcomes of a Topical Product Pre and Post Aesthetic Surgical Body Procedures. Aesthet Surg J Open Forum. 2022 Jun 10;4:ojac054. doi: 10.1093/asjof/ojac054. PMID: 35979375; PMCID: PMC9376671.

Cazzato V, Renzi N, Bottosso S, De Grazia A, Pasquali S, Di Lecce C, Martellani F, Zanconati F, Ramella V, Papa G. How Porcine Acellular Dermal Matrix Influences the Development of the Breast Capsule 1 Year after Implantation: A Histopathological Analysis. Plast Reconstr Surg Glob Open. 2023 Nov 17;11(11):e5400. doi: 10.1097/GOX.0000000000005400. PMID: 38025625; PMCID: PMC10656090.

Chatterjee SS, Khanna M. Hundred and Eleven Cases of Subfascial Breast Augmentation in Trans Women-A Single-Center Experience. Indian J Plast Surg. 2020 Mar;53(1):51-58. doi: 10.1055/s-0040-1708227. Epub 2020 Apr 17. PMID: 32367918; PMCID: PMC7192705.

Chung KJ, Park KR, Lee JH, Kim TG, Kim YH. Simvastatin Reduces Capsular Fibrosis around Silicone Implants. J Korean Med Sci. 2016 Aug;31(8):1273-8. doi: 10.3346/jkms.2016.31.8.1273. Epub 2016 May 16. Erratum in: J Korean Med Sci. 2016 Nov;31(11):1854. PMID: 27478339; PMCID: PMC4951558.

Cirocchi, R., Amabile, M.I., De Luca, A. *et al.* New classifications of axillary lymph nodes and their anatomical-clinical correlations in breast surgery. *World J Surg Onc* 19, 93 (2021). https://doi.org/10.1186/s12957-021-02209-2

Citgez B, Yigit B, Bas S. Oncoplastic and Reconstructive Breast Surgery: A Comprehensive Review. Cureus. 2022 Jan 31;14(1):e21763. doi: 10.7759/cureus.21763. PMID: 35251834; PMCID: PMC8890601.

Coady-Fariborzian L, Anstead C. Twenty Years of Breast Reduction Surgery at a Veterans Affairs Medical Center. Fed Pract. 2021 Jul;38(7):311-315. doi: 10.12788/fp.0150. PMID: 34733080; PMCID: PMC8560109.

Cohen Tervaert JW, Mohazab N, Redmond D, van Eeden C, Osman M. Breast implant illness: scientific evidence of its existence. Expert Rev Clin Immunol. 2022 Jan;18(1):15-29. doi: 10.1080/1744666X.2022.2010546. Epub 2022 Jan 5. PMID: 34882509.

Conner, K. (2023). Breast Implant Removal (Explant Surgery). Retrieved from: https://www.breastcancer.org/treatment/surgery/breast-reconstruction/types/breast-implant-removal

Cook M, Johnson N, Zegzula HD, Schray M, Glissmeyer M, Sorenson L. Prophylactic use of pentoxifylline (Trental) and vitamin E to prevent capsular contracture after implant reconstruction in patients requiring adjuvant radiation. Am J Surg. 2016 May;211(5):854-9. doi: 10.1016/j.amjsurg.2016.01.006. Epub 2016 Feb 22. PMID: 27016313.

Coombs DM, Grover R, Prassinos A, Gurunluoglu R. Breast augmentation surgery: Clinical considerations. Cleve Clin J Med. 2019 Feb;86(2):111-122. doi: 10.3949/ccjm.86a.18017. PMID: 30742581.

Cooper DC, Qureshi AA, Sharma K, Tenenbaum MM, Myckatyn TM. Impact of Breast Reconstruction Patients on Cosmetic Practice. Plast Reconstr Surg Glob Open. 2021 Jun 15;9(6):e3614. doi: 10.1097/GOX.0000000000003614. PMID: 34150419; PMCID: PMC8205214.

Davis MJ, Perdanasari AT, Abu-Ghname A, Gonzalez SR, Chamata E, Rammos CK, Winocour SJ. Application of Fat Grafting in Cosmetic Breast Surgery. Semin Plast Surg. 2020 Feb;34(1):24-29. doi: 10.1055/s-0039-1700958. Epub 2020 Feb 15. PMID: 32071576; PMCID: PMC7023973.

de Bakker, Erik MD, PhD1,2; Zada, Liron PhD3,4; Schmidt, Robert W. MSc3; van Haasterecht, Ludo MD1,3; Vethaak, A. Dick PhD4,5; Ariese, Freek PhD3; Dijkman, Henry B. P. M. PhD6; Bult, Peter MD, PhD7; Gibbs, Susan PhD2,8; Niessen, Frank B. MD, PhD1. Baker Grade IV Capsular Contracture Is Correlated with an Increased Amount of Silicone Material: An Intrapatient Study. Plastic and

Reconstructive Surgery 152(6):p 1191-1200, December 2023. | DOI: 10.1097/PRS.0000000000010359

DePolo, J. (2023). Types of Breast Reconstruction Procedures. Retrieved from: https://www.breastcancer.org/treatment/surgery/breast-reconstruction/types

De Vrieze T, Gebruers N, Nevelsteen I, Fieuws S, Thomis S, De Groef A, Tjalma WA, Belgrado JP, Vandermeeren L, Monten C, Hanssens M, Devoogdt N. Manual lymphatic drainage with or without fluoroscopy guidance did not substantially improve the effect of decongestive lymphatic therapy in people with breast cancer-related lymphoedema (EFforT-BCRL trial): a multicentre randomised trial. J Physiother. 2022 Apr;68(2):110-122. doi: 10.1016/j.jphys.2022.03.010. Epub 2022 Apr 12. PMID: 35428594.

Dilaveri CA, Croghan IT, Mallory MJ, Dion LJ, Fischer KM, Schroeder DR, Martinez-Jorge J, Nguyen MT, Fokken SC, Bauer BA, Wahner-Roedler DL. Massage Compared with Massage Plus Acupuncture for Breast Cancer Patients Undergoing Reconstructive Surgery. J Altern Complement Med. 2020 Jul;26(7):602-609. doi: 10.1089/acm.2019.0479. PMID: 32673082; PMCID: PMC7374617.

Dion LJ, Engen DJ, Lemaine V, Lawson DK, Brock CG, Thomley BS, Cha SS, Sood A, Bauer BA, Wahner-Roedler DL. Massage therapy alone and in combination with meditation for breast cancer patients undergoing autologous tissue reconstruction: A randomized pilot study. Complement Ther Clin Pract. 2016 May;23:82-7. doi: 10.1016/j.ctcp.2015.04.005. Epub 2015 May 12. PMID: 25986296.

Dixit, V. V., & Wagh, M. S. (2013). Unfavourable outcomes of liposuction and their management. *Indian Journal of Plastic Surgery*, 46(2), 377–92.

Dong, Chen MD; Yu, Zhou MD, PhD; Du, Jing MD; Zhang, Yu MD; Liu, Wei MD; Huang, Zhaosong MD; Xiong, Shaoheng MD; Wang, Tong MD; Song, Yajuan MD; Ma, Xianjie MD, PhD. Montelukast Attenuates Retraction of Expanded Flap by Inhibiting Capsule Formation around Silicone Expander through TGF-β1 Signaling. Plastic and Reconstructive Surgery 152(6):p 1044e-1052e, December 2023. | DOI: 10.1097/PRS.0000000000010459

Drackley NL, Degnim AC, Jakub JW, Cutshall SM, Thomley BS, Brodt JK, Vanderlei LK, Case JK, Bungum LD, Cha SS, Bauer BA, Boughey JC. Effect of massage therapy for postsurgical mastectomy recipients. Clin J Oncol Nurs. 2012 Apr;16(2):121-4. doi: 10.1188/12.CJON.121-124. PMID: 22459520.

Edinoff AN, Raveendran K, Colon MA, Thomas BH, Trettin KA, Hunt GW, Kaye AM, Cornett EM, Kaye AD. Selective Serotonin Reuptake Inhibitors and Associated Bleeding Risks: A Narrative and Clinical Review. Health Psychol Res. 2022 Nov 3;10(4):39580. doi: 10.52965/001c.39580. PMID: 36425234; PMCID: PMC9680839.

Elahi L, Meuwly MG, Meuwly JY, Raffoul W, Koch N. Management of Contralateral Breast and Axillary Nodes Silicone Migration after Implant Rupture. Plast Reconstr Surg Glob Open. 2022 May 25;10(5):e4290. doi: 10.1097/GOX.0000000000004290. PMID: 35646497; PMCID: PMC9132530.

Fat Grafting and Lipofilling (2024). Retrieved from: https://www.reclaimyourcurves.org.au/fat-grafting.html

FDA Updates Analysis of Medical Device Reports of Breast Implant Illness and Breast Implant-Associated Lymphoma. Accessed August 20, 2020. https://www.fda.gov/news-events/press-announcements/fda-updates-analysis-medical-device-reports-breast-implant-illness-and-breast-implant-associated.

Figus A, Mazzocchi M, Dessy LA, Curinga G, Scuderi N. Treatment of muscular contraction deformities with botulinum toxin type A after latissimus dorsi flap and sub-pectoral implant breast reconstruction. J Plast Reconstr Aesthet Surg. 2009 Jul;62(7):869-75. doi: 10.1016/j.bjps.2007.07.025. Epub 2008 Apr 14. PMID: 18411075.

Flores T, Kerschbaumer C, Jaklin FJ, Rohrbacher A, Weber M, Luft M, Aspöck C, Ströbele B, Kitzwögerer M, Lumenta DB, Bergmeister KD, Schrögendorfer KF. Gram-Positive Bacteria Increase Breast Implant-Related Complications: Prospective Analysis of 100 Revised Implants. Plast Reconstr Surg. 2024 Jan 1;153(1):76-89. doi: 10.1097/PRS.0000000000010499. Epub 2023 Apr 11. PMID: 37036325; PMCID: PMC10729897.

Földi E, Földi M, (eds) (2012) Textbook of lymphology. Munich: Urban & Fischer.

Fontes, Tomás & Brandão, Inês & Negrão, Rita & Martins, Maria João & Monteiro, Rosário. (2018). Autologous fat grafting: Harvesting techniques. Annals of Medicine and Surgery. 36. 10.1016/j.amsu.2018.11.005.

Fracol M, Feld LN, Chiu WK, Kim JYS. An overview of animation deformity in prosthetic breast reconstruction. Gland Surg. 2019 Feb;8(1):95-101. doi: 10.21037/gs.2018.09.09. PMID: 30842934; PMCID: PMC6378247.

Fusaro M, Bufacchi RJ, Nicolardi V, Provenzano L. The analgesic power of pleasant touch in individuals with chronic pain: Recent findings and new insights. Front Integr Neurosci. 2022 Sep 13;16:956510. doi: 10.3389/fnint.2022.956510. PMID: 36176327; PMCID: PMC9513358.

Gabriel A, Champaneria MC, Maxwell GP. Fat grafting and breast reconstruction: tips for ensuring predictability. Gland Surg. 2015 Jun;4(3):232-43. doi: 10.3978/j.issn.2227-684X.2015.04.18. PMID: 26161308; PMCID: PMC4461705.

Gabriel A, Champaneria MC, Maxwell GP. The efficacy of botulinum toxin A in post-mastectomy breast reconstruction: a pilot study. Aesthet Surg J. 2015 May;35(4):402-9. doi: 10.1093/asj/sjv040. Epub 2015 Mar 29. PMID: 25825421.

Gao Y, Shang Q, Li W, Guo W, Stojadinovic A, Mannion C, Man YG, Chen T. Antibiotics for cancer treatment: A double-edged sword. J Cancer. 2020 Jun 28;11(17):5135-5149. doi: 10.7150/jca.47470. PMID: 32742461; PMCID: PMC7378927.

Gargano F, Ciminello F, Podda S, De Santis G. Salvage of exposed breast implant using capsular flaps. Eplasty. 2009 Sep 17;9:e41. PMID: 19838292; PMCID: PMC2752472.

Gerzenshtein, Jacob M.D.. The Dishonesty of Referring to Total Intact Capsulectomy as "En Bloc" Resection or Capsulectomy. Plastic and Reconstructive Surgery 145(1):p 227e-228e, January 2020. | DOI: 10.1097/PRS.0000000000006362

Giometti MCS, Sobral CS, Abdala J, Gomes DT. Comparison of anatomic and round implants using periareolar access in primary breast augmentation. Rev. Bras. Cir. Plást.2016;31(3):328-338

Graziano, Francis D. MD; Plotsker, Ethan L. BA; Rubenstein, Robyn N. MD; Haglich, Kathryn MS; Stern, Carrie S. MD; Matros, Evan MD, MPH, MMSc; Nelson, Jonas A. MD, MPH. National Trends in Acellular Dermal Matrix Utilization in Immediate Breast Reconstruction. Plastic and Reconstructive Surgery 153(1):p 25e-36e, January 2024. | DOI: 10.1097/PRS.0000000000010575

Greenbaum A, Halpert G, Dotan A, Shivatzki S, Heidecke H, Kaplan Neeman R, Ehrenfeld M, Wolfovitz A, Amital H, Henkin Y, Shoenfeld Y. The Prevalence of Hearing Impairments in Women with Silicone Breast Implants. Diseases. 2023 Feb 9;11(1):31. doi: 10.3390/diseases11010031. PMID: 36810545; PMCID: PMC9945132.

Gerzenshtein, Jacob M.D.. The Dishonesty of Referring to Total Intact Capsulectomy as "En Bloc" Resection or Capsulectomy. Plastic and Reconstructive Surgery 145(1):p 227e-228e, January 2020. | DOI: 10.1097/PRS.0000000000006362

Gilfillan AM, Austin SJ, Metcalfe DD. Mast cell biology: introduction and overview. Adv Exp Med Biol. 2011;716:2-12. doi: 10.1007/978-1-4419-9533-9_1. PMID: 21713648; PMCID: PMC3398748.

Guimier E, Carson L, David B, Lambert JM, Heery E, Malcolm RK. Pharmacological Approaches for the Prevention of Breast Implant Capsular Contracture. J Surg Res. 2022 Dec;280:129-150. doi: 10.1016/j.jss.2022.06.073. Epub 2022 Aug 12. PMID: 35969932.

Hansen TC, Woeller CF, Lacy SH, Koltz PF, Langstein HN, Phipps RP. Thy1 (CD90) Expression Is Elevated in Radiation-Induced Periprosthetic Capsular Contracture: Implication for Novel Therapeutics. Plast Reconstr Surg. 2017 Aug;140(2):316-326. doi: 10.1097/PRS.0000000000003542. PMID: 28746279; PMCID: PMC5531053.

Harlim A, Kanoko M, Aisah S. Classification of Foreign Body Reactions due to Industrial Silicone Injection. Dermatol Surg. 2018

Sep;44(9):1174-1182. doi: 10.1097/DSS.0000000000001531. PMID: 29757858; PMCID: PMC6112849.

Hauch AT, Francis CS, Artz JD, Chasan PE. Subpectoral Implant Repositioning With Partial Capsule Preservation: Treating the Long-Term Complications of Subglandular Breast Augmentation. Aesthet Surg J Open Forum. 2021 Mar 2;3(2):ojab009. doi: 10.1093/asjof/ojab009. PMID: 34212143; PMCID: PMC8240740.

Holistic Accelerated Recovery Program (n.d.) Retrieved from: https://www.drrobertwhitfield.com/bii-recovery/

Hope J. A review of the mechanism of injury and treatment approaches for illness resulting from exposure to water-damaged buildings, mold, and mycotoxins. ScientificWorldJournal. 2013 Apr 18;2013:767482. doi: 10.1155/2013/767482. PMID: 23710148; PMCID: PMC3654247.

How do breasts look after explant surgery (n.d.). Retrieved from: https://www.timsayedmd.com/how-do-breasts-look-after-explant-surgery/

Huang CK, Handel N. Effects of Singulair (montelukast) treatment for capsular contracture. Aesthet Surg J. 2010 May-Jun;30(3):404-8. doi: 10.1177/1090820X10374724. PMID: 20601564.

Jones HE, Faulkner HR, Losken A. The Psychological Impact of Aesthetic Surgery: A Mini-Review. Aesthet Surg J Open Forum. 2022 Oct 13;4:ojac077. doi: 10.1093/asjof/ojac077. PMID: 36447649; PMCID: PMC9687813.

Jud SM, Brendle-Behnisch A, Hack CC, Preuss C, Arkudas A, Horch RE, Beckmann MW, Lux MP. Macromastia: an economic burden? A disease cost analysis based on real-world data in Germany. Arch Gynecol Obstet. 2021 Feb;303(2):521-531. doi: 10.1007/s00404-020-05841-7. Epub 2020 Oct 29. PMID: 33123809; PMCID: PMC7858209.

Kalaria SS, Henderson J, Moliver CL. Iatrogenic Symmastia: Causes and Suggested Repair Technique. Aesthet Surg J. 2019 Jul 12;39(8):863-872. doi: 10.1093/asj/sjy217. PMID: 30137185.

Katsnelson, Jacob Y. MD*; Spaniol, Joseph R. MD†; Buinewicz, Joshua C. BA‡; Ramsey, Frederick V. PhD§; Buinewicz, Brian R. MD, FACS*,‡. Outcomes of Implant Removal and Capsulectomy for Breast Implant Illness in 248 Patients. Plastic and Reconstructive Surgery - Global Open 9(9):p e3813, September 2021. | DOI: 10.1097/GOX.0000000000003813

Kehlet H, Dahl JB. Anaesthesia, surgery, and challenges in postoperative recovery. Lancet. 2003 Dec 6;362(9399):1921-8. doi: 10.1016/S0140-6736(03)14966-5. PMID: 14667752.

Kennedy L, Sandhu JK, Harper ME, Cuperlovic-Culf M. Role of Glutathione in Cancer: From Mechanisms to Therapies. Biomolecules. 2020 Oct 9;10(10):1429. doi: 10.3390/biom10101429. PMID: 33050144; PMCID: PMC7600400.

Kerr F, Wiechula R, Feo R, Schultz T, Kitson A. Neurophysiology of human touch and eye gaze in therapeutic relationships and healing: a scoping review. JBI Database System Rev Implement Rep. 2019 Feb;17(2):209-247. doi: 10.11124/JBISRIR-2017-003549. PMID: 30730854; PMCID: PMC6382052.

Keser I, Esmer M. Does Manual Lymphatic Drainage Have Any Effect on Pain Threshold and Tolerance of Different Body Parts? Lymphat Res Biol. 2019 Dec;17(6):651-654. doi: 10.1089/lrb.2019.0005. Epub 2019 Jul 19. PMID: 31329499.

Kim JH, Lee S, Najmiddinov B, Kim EK, Myung Y, Heo CY. Risk factors for chest wall depression after implant insertion for breast reconstruction: a retrospective quantitative study. Gland Surg. 2022 Aug;11(8):1333-1340. doi: 10.21037/gs-22-101. PMID: 36082096; PMCID: PMC9445711.

Kim SJ, Kwon OY, Yi CH. Effects of manual lymph drainage on cardiac autonomic tone in healthy subjects. Int J Neurosci. 2009;119(8):1105-17. doi: 10.1080/00207450902834884. PMID: 19922342.

Kim M, Ali B, Ly C, Zhang K, Boe L, Stern CS, Allen RJ Jr, Matros E, Nelson JA, Mehrara BJ. Using the 5-Item Modified Frailty Index to Predict Breast-Q Scores— an Analysis of 2,160 Autologous Breast

Reconstruction Patients. Plast Reconstr Surg Glob Open. 2024 Jan 8;12(1 Suppl):36. doi: 10.1097/01.GOX.0001006040.31071.56. PMCID: PMC10775221.

Kim, Y. H., Yang, Y. J., Lee, D. W., Song, S. Y., Lew, D. H., & Yang, E. J. Prevention of postoperative complications by prepectoral versus subpectoral breast reconstruction: A systematic review and meta-analysis. *Plastic and Reconstructive Surgery*, 10-1097.

Kirby RM, Basit A, Nguyen QT, Jaipersad A, Billingham R. Three stage axillary lymphatic massage optimizes sentinel lymph node localisation using blue dye. Int Semin Surg Oncol. 2007 Dec 22;4:30. doi: 10.1186/1477-7800-4-30. PMID: 18154682; PMCID: PMC2248582.

Klose, G. (2014 Oct. 1) How manual lymph drainage certification will change your massage practice. Retrieved from https://www.massagemag.com/how-manual-lymph-drainage-certification-will-change-your-massage-practice-27028.

Ko, M. (2021). The Effect of Manual Lymphatic Drainage on the Stress and Pain in Patient with Postoperative Breast Cancer. *Physical Therapy Rehabilitation Science*.

la Fleur P, Adams A. Botulinum Toxin for Temporomandibular Disorders: A Review of Clinical Effectiveness, Cost-Effectiveness, and Guidelines [Internet]. Ottawa (ON): Canadian Agency for Drugs and Technologies in Health; 2020 Feb 25. PMID: 33074614.

Lampert JA, Townsend AN, Shah S, Bouz A, Nichols N. Safely Shaping the Breast After Implant Removal and Total Intact Capsulectomy Using the Mammary Imbrication Lift and Fixation Technique. Aesthet Surg J Open Forum. 2023 Apr 12;5:ojad037. doi: 10.1093/asjof/ojad037. PMID: 37228315; PMCID: PMC10205400.

Larsen A, Rasmussen LE, Rasmussen LF, Weltz TK, Hemmingsen MN, Poulsen SS, Jacobsen JCB, Vester-Glowinski P, Herly M. Histological Analyses of Capsular Contracture and Associated Risk Factors: A Systematic Review. Aesthetic Plast Surg. 2021 Dec;45(6):2714-2728. doi: 10.1007/s00266-021-02473-3. Epub 2021 Jul 26. PMID: 34312696.

Lee M, Ponraja G, McLeod K, Chong S. Breast Implant Illness: A Biofilm Hypothesis. Plast Reconstr Surg Glob Open. 2020 Apr 30;8(4):e2755. doi: 10.1097/GOX.0000000000002755. PMID: 32440423; PMCID: PMC7209857.

Le Louarn C, Buis J, Auclair E. Flector tissugel used to treat capsular contracture after breast augmentation surgery. Aesthetic Plast Surg. 2008 May;32(3):453-8. doi: 10.1007/s00266-008-9123-0. PMID: 18389304.

Lieffering AS, Hommes JE, Ramerman L, Rakhorst HA, Mureau MAM, Verheij RA, van der Hulst RRWJ. Prevalence of Local Postoperative Complications and Breast Implant Illness in Women With Breast Implants. JAMA Netw Open. 2022 Oct 3;5(10):e2236519. doi: 10.1001/jamanetworkopen.2022.36519. PMID: 36205992; PMCID: PMC9547313.

Liu H, Akhavan A, Yin R, Ibelli T, Mandelbaum M, Katz A, Etigunta S, Alerte E, Kuruvilla A, Liu C, Taub PJ. Efficacy of the Modified 5-Item Frailty Index in Predicting Surgical-Site Infections in Patients Undergoing Breast Implant Augmentation: A National Surgical Quality Improvement Project-Based 5-Year Study. Aesthet Surg J Open Forum. 2023 Jul 18;5:ojad067. doi: 10.1093/asjof/ojad067. PMID: 37575888; PMCID: PMC10413997.

Lombardo GAG, Tamburino S, Magano K, Fagone P, Mammana S, Cavalli E, Basile MS, Salvatorelli L, Catalano F, Magro G, Nicoletti F. The Effect of Omega-3 Fatty Acids on Capsular Tissue around the Breast Implants. Plast Reconstr Surg. 2020 Mar;145(3):701-710. doi: 10.1097/PRS.0000000000006553. PMID: 32097310.

Lonie S, Sachs R, Shen A, Hunter-Smith DJ, Rozen WM, Seifman M. A systematic review of patient reported outcome measures for women with macromastia who have undergone breast reduction surgery. Gland Surg. 2019 Aug;8(4):431-440. doi: 10.21037/gs.2019.03.08. PMID: 31538069; PMCID: PMC6722998.

Lubczyńska A, Garncarczyk A, Wcisło-Dziadecka D. Effectiveness of various methods of manual scar therapy. Skin Res Technol. 2023 Mar;29(3):e13272. doi: 10.1111/srt.13272. PMID: 36973982; PMCID: PMC10155853.

Lymphatic Drainage Massage (2021). Retrieved from: https://my.clevelandclinic.org/health/treatments/21768-lymphatic-drainage-massage

McConnell JP, Moyer TP, Nixon DE, Schnur PL, Salomao DR, Crotty TB, Weinzweig J, Harris JB, Petty PM. Determination of silicon in breast and capsular tissue from patients with breast implants performed by inductively coupled plasma emission spectroscopy. Comparison with tissue histology. Am J Clin Pathol. 1997 Feb;107(2):236-46. doi: 10.1093/ajcp/107.2.236. PMID: 9024074.

McNemar, T., Salzberg, C. A., & Seidel, S. (2006). *Breast augmentation and body contouring*. Omaha, NE: Addicus Books.

Martinez CA, Boutros SG. Abdominoplasty and Breast Augmentation with Outpatient Cosmetic Deep Inferior Epigastric Perforator Flaps. Plast Reconstr Surg. 2023 Feb 1;151(2):234e-240e. doi: 10.1097/PRS.0000000000009836. Epub 2022 Nov 11. PMID: 36354968.

Marwa K, Anjum F. Undifferentiated Connective Tissue Disease. [Updated 2023 Apr 27]. In: StatPearls [Internet]. Treasure Island (FL): StatPearls Publishing; 2023 Jan-.

Marxen T, Shauly O, Goel P, Tsan T, Faria R, Gould DJ. The Utility of Lymphatic Massage in Cosmetic Procedures. Aesthet Surg J Open Forum. 2023 Feb 28;5:ojad023. doi: 10.1093/asjof/ojad023. PMID: 36998743; PMCID: PMC10045879.

Massage Therapy Act 2023 (2023). Retrieved from: https://www.camtc.org/media/2249/massage-therapy-act-2023.pdf

Massingill J, Jorgensen C, Dolata J, Sehgal AR. Myofascial Massage for Chronic Pain and Decreased Upper Extremity Mobility After Breast Cancer Surgery. Int J Ther Massage Bodywork. 2018 Aug 5;11(3):4-9. PMID: 30108667; PMCID: PMC6087660.

Mazuquin B, Sunemi MMO, E Silva MPP, Sarian LOZ, Williamson E, Bruce J. Current physical therapy care of patients undergoing breast reconstruction for breast cancer: a survey of practice in the United Kingdom and Brazil. Braz J Phys Ther. 2021 Mar-

Apr;25(2):175-185. doi: 10.1016/j.bjpt.2020.05.010. Epub 2020 Jun 4. PMID: 32605886; PMCID: PMC7990737.

Menard MB. Immediate Effect of Therapeutic Massage on Pain Sensation and Unpleasantness: A Consecutive Case Series. Glob Adv Health Med. 2015 Sep;4(5):56-60. doi: 10.7453/gahmj.2015.059. Epub 2015 Sep 1. PMID: 26421235; PMCID: PMC4563896.

Metzinger SE, Homsy C, Chun MJ, Metzinger RC. Breast Implant Illness: Treatment Using Total Capsulectomy and Implant Removal. Eplasty. 2022 Mar 16;22:e5. PMID: 35602522; PMCID: PMC9097901.

Miller, C.S., Palmer, R.F., Dempsey, T.T. *et al.* Mast cell activation may explain many cases of chemical intolerance. *Environ Sci Eur* 33, 129 (2021). https://doi.org/10.1186/s12302-021-00570-3

Miozzo AP, Stein C, Bozzetto CB, Plentz RD. Massage therapy reduces pain and anxiety after cardiac surgery: A systematic review and meta-analysis of randomized clinical trials. *Clin Trials Regul Sci Cardiol* 2016;23:1–8.

Mohan, Abee S. MD, PhD1; Sullivan, Janessa BA2; Tenenbaum, Marissa M. MD2; Broderick, Kristen B. MD1; Myckatyn, Terence M. MD2. Toward a Consensus Approach for Assessing Capsular Contracture Severity and Progression: A Systematic Review. Plastic and Reconstructive Surgery 153(1):p 7-22, January 2024. | DOI: 10.1097/PRS.0000000000010573

Mowlavi A, Asghari A, Heydarlou D, Gavilanes E, Sin Z, Mirzania H. Breast Lift Algorithm for the Treatment of Breast Implant Illness Requiring Implant Removal. Aesthetic Plast Surg. 2023 Jun;47(3):934-943. doi: 10.1007/s00266-022-03178-x. Epub 2022 Nov 22. PMID: 36414723.

Nava, Maurizio & Blondeel, Phillip & Botti, Giovanni & Casabona, Francesco & Catanuto, Giuseppe & Clemens, Mark & Fazio, Domenico & Vita, Roy & Grotting, James & Hammond, Dennis & Harris, Paul & Montemurro, Paolo & Mendonça Munhoz, Alexandre & Nahabedian, Maurice & Pompei, Stefano & Rancati, Alberto & Rigotti, Gino & Salgarello, Marzia & Scaperrotta, Gianfranco & Rocco, Nicola. (2019). International Expert Panel Consensus on Fat

Grafting of the Breast. Plastic and Reconstructive Surgery - Global Open. 7. 1. 10.1097/GOX.0000000000002426.

Nevola Teixeira, Luiz Felipe & Sandrin, Fabio. (2014). The role of the physiotherapy in the plastic surgery patients after oncological breast surgery. Gland Surgery. 3. 43-47. 10.3978/j.issn.2227-684X.2014.02.12.

Nicoloro-SantaBarbara J, Carroll J, Lobel M. Coping, social support, and anxiety in people with mast cell disorders. Ann Allergy Asthma Immunol. 2021 Oct;127(4):435-440. doi: 10.1016/j.anai.2021.06.014. Epub 2021 Jun 19. PMID: 34153442; PMCID: PMC9909465.

Papaconstantinou A, Koletsa T, Demiri E, et al. Nonsurgical treatment of capsular contracture: Review of clinical studies. Journal of International Medical Research. 2020;48(6). doi:10.1177/0300060520927873

Oncology Massage Therapy Guidelines—Safe and Beneficial at all Stages of Cancer (2023). Retrieved from: https://www.s4om.org/wp-content/uploads/2023/12/S4OM-Position-Paper-Oncology-Massage-Therapy-Guidelines%E2%80%94Safe-and-Beneficial-at-all-Stages-of-Cancer-12.2023.pdf

Opett, A. (n.d.). Medbridge class 'Tissue Injury: Mechanisms of Inflammation and Repair.' Retrieved from: https://www.medbridgeeducation.com/course-catalog/details/tissue-injury-mechanisms-inflammation-repair-andrew-opett/

ORDINANCE NO. 10102 (N.S.) (2010). Retrieved from: https://www.sandiegocounty.gov/content/dam/sdc/cob/ordinances/ord10102.doc

Patel A, Blackmore K, Carruthers R. The Integrated Treatment for Chronic Pain and Anxiety in a Patient with Breast Implant Illness Symptoms: A Case Report. Integr Med (Encinitas). 2020 Aug;19(4):28-33. PMID: 33132782; PMCID: PMC7572138.

Paul S, Chakraborty S, Anand U, Dey S, Nandy S, Ghorai M, Saha SC, Patil MT, Kandimalla R, Proćków J, Dey A. Withania somnifera (L.) Dunal (Ashwagandha): A comprehensive review on ethnopharmacology, pharmacotherapeutics, biomedicinal and toxicological aspects. Biomed Pharmacother. 2021 Nov;143:112175. doi: 10.1016/j.biopha.2021.112175. Epub 2021 Sep 27. PMID: 34649336.

PDQ Integrative, Alternative, and Complementary Therapies Editorial Board. Milk Thistle (PDQ®): Health Professional Version. 2022 Feb 17. In: PDQ Cancer Information Summaries [Internet]. Bethesda (MD): National Cancer Institute (US); 2002–. PMID: 26389223.

Portillo ME, Corvec S, Borens O, Trampuz A. Propionibacterium acnes: an underestimated pathogen in implant-associated infections. Biomed Res Int. 2013;2013:804391. doi: 10.1155/2013/804391. Epub 2013 Nov 6. PMID: 24308006; PMCID: PMC3838805.

Qi D, Liu Y, Li J, Huang JH, Hu X, Wu E. Salinomycin as a potent anticancer stem cell agent: State of the art and future directions. Med Res Rev. 2022 May;42(3):1037-1063. doi: 10.1002/med.21870. Epub 2021 Nov 16. PMID: 34786735; PMCID: PMC9298915.

Raghu G, Berk M, Campochiaro PA, Jaeschke H, Marenzi G, Richeldi L, Wen FQ, Nicoletti F, Calverley PMA. The Multifaceted Therapeutic Role of N-Acetylcysteine (NAC) in Disorders Characterized by Oxidative Stress. Curr Neuropharmacol. 2021;19(8):1202-1224. doi: 10.2174/1570159X19666201230144109. PMID: 33380301; PMCID: PMC8719286.

Rajgor AD, Mentias Y, Stafford F. Silicone granuloma: a cause of cervical lymphadenopathy following breast implantation. BMJ Case Rep. 2021 Mar 3;14(3):e239395. doi: 10.1136/bcr-2020-239395. PMID: 33658215; PMCID: PMC7931750.

Ramanadham SR, Rose Johnson A. Breast Lift with and without Implant: A Synopsis and Primer for the Plastic Surgeon. Plast Reconstr Surg Glob Open. 2020 Oct 28;8(10):e3057. doi: 10.1097/GOX.0000000000003057. PMID: 33173660; PMCID: PMC7647657.

Ramirez J, Guarner F, Bustos Fernandez L, Maruy A, Sdepanian VL, Cohen H. Antibiotics as Major Disruptors of Gut Microbiota.

Front Cell Infect Microbiol. 2020 Nov 24;10:572912. doi: 10.3389/fcimb.2020.572912. PMID: 33330122; PMCID: PMC7732679.

Rand, R. (2019 Jan. 15). What is an auto-augmentation breast lift? Retrieved from: https://www.plasticsurgery.org/news/blog/what-is-an-auto-augmentation-breast-lift

Rapaport MH, Schettler P, Breese C. A preliminary study of the effects of a single session of Swedish massage on hypothalamic-pituitary-adrenal and immune function in normal individuals. J Altern Complement Med. 2010 Oct;16(10):1079-88. doi: 10.1089/acm.2009.0634. PMID: 20809811; PMCID: PMC3107905.

Ratz-Łyko A, Arct J, Pytkowska K. Moisturizing and Antiinflammatory Properties of Cosmetic Formulations Containing Centella asiatica Extract. Indian J Pharm Sci. 2016 Jan-Feb;78(1):27-33. doi: 10.4103/0250-474x.180247. PMID: 27168678; PMCID: PMC4852572.

Rinaldi RM, Sapra A, Bellin LS. Breast Lymphatics. [Updated 2023 Aug 8]. In: StatPearls [Internet]. Treasure Island (FL): StatPearls Publishing; 2023 Jan-.

Risks and complications of breast implants (2023). Retrieved from: https://www.fda.gov/medical-devices/breast-implants/risks-and-complications-breast-implants

Schoffer AK, Bittner AK, Hess J, Kimmig R, Hoffmann O. Complications and satisfaction in transwomen receiving breast augmentation: short- and long-term outcomes. Arch Gynecol Obstet. 2022 Jun;305(6):1517-1524. doi: 10.1007/s00404-022-06603-3. Epub 2022 May 21. PMID: 35597817; PMCID: PMC9166844.

Sevick-Muraca EM, Fife CE, Rasmussen JC. Imaging peripheral lymphatic dysfunction in chronic conditions. Front Physiol. 2023 Mar 15;14:1132097. doi: 10.3389/fphys.2023.1132097. PMID: 37007996; PMCID: PMC10050385.

Sheng, L., Yu, Q., Xie, F., & Li, Q. (2014). Foreign body response induced by tissue expander implantation. Molecular Medicine Reports, 9, 872-876. https://doi.org/10.3892/mmr.2013.1881

Schwartz N, Chalasani MLS, Li TM, Feng Z, Shipman WD, Lu TT. Lymphatic Function in Autoimmune Diseases. Front Immunol. 2019 Mar 20;10:519. doi: 10.3389/fimmu.2019.00519. PMID: 30949174; PMCID: PMC6435962.

Silverstein, Max L. MD1; Momeni, Arash MD2. Long-Term Outcomes Following Hybrid Breast Reconstruction. Plastic & Reconstructive Surgery-Global Open 12(1S1):p 9, January 2024. | DOI: 10.1097/01.GOX.0001005876.78580.46

Sinno, S., & Hidalgo, D. (2016). Abstract: Current Trends and Controversies in Breast Augmentation. *Plastic and Reconstructive Surgery Global Open*, *4*(9 Suppl), 136-137. https://doi.org/10.1097/01.GOX.0000503061.17309.3d

Sobti, N., Weitzman, R.E., Nealon, K.P. *et al.* Evaluation of capsular contracture following immediate prepectoral versus subpectoral direct-to-implant breast reconstruction. *Sci Rep* 10, 1137 (2020). https://doi.org/10.1038/s41598-020-58094-4

Søndergaard S. Observational study on passive leg raising and the autonomic nervous system. Physiol Rep. 2022 Dec;10(24):e15537. doi: 10.14814/phy2.15537. PMID: 36541245; PMCID: PMC9768665.

Sood A, Xue EY, Sangiovanni C, Therattil PJ, Lee ES. Breast Massage, Implant Displacement, and Prevention of Capsular Contracture After Breast Augmentation With Implants: A Review of the Literature. Eplasty. 2017 Dec 21;17:e41. PMID: 29348783; PMCID: PMC5749369.

Stamouli A, Lanitis S, Kontos M. Pectoralis Major Muscle Morbidity After Submuscular Silicone-based Breast Reconstruction: A Systematic Review. In Vivo. 2023 Sep-Oct;37(5):1931-1939. doi: 10.21873/invivo.13289. PMID: 37652471; PMCID: PMC10500532.

Standards of Practice (2017) Retrieved from: https://www.ncbtmb.org/standards-of-practice/

Stümpfle RL, Piccinini PS, Zanin EM. Transabdominal Breast Augmentation With Silicone Gel Implants. Ann Plast Surg. 2021 Aug 1;87(2):126-131. doi: 10.1097/SAP.0000000000002921. PMID: 34176905.

Susini P, Nisi G, Pierazzi DM, Giardino FR, Pozzi M, Grimaldi L, Cuomo R. Advances on Capsular Contracture-Prevention and Management Strategies: A Narrative Review of the Literature. Plast Reconstr Surg Glob Open. 2023 Jun 9;11(6):e5034. doi: 10.1097/GOX.0000000000005034. PMID: 37305202; PMCID: PMC10256414.

Swezey E, Shikhman R, Moufarrege R. Breast Implant Rupture. 2023 Jan 16. In: StatPearls [Internet]. Treasure Island (FL): StatPearls Publishing; 2023 Jan–. PMID: 29083733.

Ucuzal M, Kanan N. Foot massage: effectiveness on postoperative pain in breast surgery patients. Pain Manag Nurs. 2014 Jun;15(2):458-65. doi: 10.1016/j.pmn.2012.03.001. Epub 2012 Jun 20. PMID: 24882025.

Van Boerum MS, Salibian AA, Bluebond-Langner R, Agarwal C. Chest and facial surgery for the transgender patient. Transl Androl Urol. 2019 Jun;8(3):219-227. doi: 10.21037/tau.2019.06.18. PMID: 31380228; PMCID: PMC6626311.

Veras-Castillo ER, Cardenas-Camarena L, Lyra-Gonzalez I, Muñoz-Valle JF, Lucano-Landeros S, Guerrerosantos J, Gonzalez-Ulloa B, Mercado-Barajas JL, Sanchez-Parada MG, Azabache-Wennceslao R, Armendariz-Borunda J. Controlled clinical trial with pirfenidone in the treatment of breast capsular contracture: association of TGF-β polymorphisms. Ann Plast Surg. 2013 Jan;70(1):16-22. doi: 10.1097/SAP.0b013e31822284f4. PMID: 21712700.

Vairo GL, Miller SJ, McBrier NM, Buckley WE. Systematic review of efficacy for manual lymphatic drainage techniques in sports medicine and rehabilitation: an evidence-based practice approach. J Man Manip Ther. 2009;17(3):e80-9. doi: 10.1179/jmt.2009.17.3.80E. PMID: 20046617; PMCID: PMC2755111.

Vidya R, Iqbal FM, Becker H, Zhadan O. Rippling Associated with Pre-Pectoral Implant Based Breast Reconstruction: A New Grading System. World J Plast Surg. 2019 Sep;8(3):311-315. doi: 10.29252/wjps.8.3.311. PMID: 31620332; PMCID: PMC6790253.

Wagner RD, Lisiecki JL, Chiodo MV, Rohrich RJ. Longevity of ptosis correction in mastopexy and reduction mammaplasty: A systematic review of techniques. JPRAS Open. 2022 May 13;34:1-9. doi: 10.1016/j.jpra.2022.05.003. PMID: 36061406; PMCID: PMC9428726.

Wang Y, Tian J, Liu J. Suppressive Effect of Leukotriene Antagonists on Capsular Contracture in Patients Who Underwent Breast Surgery with Prosthesis: A Meta-Analysis. Plast Reconstr Surg. 2020 Apr;145(4):901-911. doi: 10.1097/PRS.0000000000006629. PMID: 32221199.

Wang R, Huang X, Wang Y, Akbari M. Non-pharmacologic Approaches in Preoperative Anxiety, a Comprehensive Review. Front Public Health. 2022 Apr 11;10:854673. doi: 10.3389/fpubh.2022.854673. PMID: 35480569; PMCID: PMC9035831.

Watad A, Quaresma M, Bragazzi NL, Cervera R, Tervaert JWC, Amital H, Shoenfeld Y. The autoimmune/inflammatory syndrome induced by adjuvants (ASIA)/Shoenfeld's syndrome: descriptive analysis of 300 patients from the international ASIA syndrome registry. Clin Rheumatol. 2018 Feb;37(2):483-493. doi: 10.1007/s10067-017-3748-9. Epub 2017 Jul 25. PMID: 28741088.

Watson S, Kaminsky E, Taavola H, Attalla M, Yue QY. Montelukast and Nightmares: Further Characterisation Using Data from VigiBase. Drug Saf. 2022 Jun;45(6):675-684. doi: 10.1007/s40264-022-01183-2. Epub 2022 Jun 1. PMID: 35650509; PMCID: PMC9189082. Retrieved from: Watson S, Kaminsky E, Taavola H, Attalla M, Yue QY. Montelukast and Nightmares: Further Characterisation Using Data from VigiBase. Drug Saf. 2022 Jun;45(6):675-684. doi: 10.1007/s40264-022-01183-2. Epub 2022 Jun 1. PMID: 35650509; PMCID: PMC9189082.

White CP, Peterson BD. Augmentation Mastopexy with Surgical Excision of the Lower Pole to Avoid Waterfall Deformity: A Surgical Technique and Nipple Areolar Complex Case Series. Plast Surg (Oakv). 2021 May;29(2):103-109. doi: 10.1177/2292550320933662. Epub 2020 Jul 21. Erratum in: Plast Surg (Oakv). 2021 Nov;29(4):303. PMID: 34026673; PMCID: PMC8120554.

Williams A. Manual lymphatic drainage: exploring the history and evidence base. Br J Community Nurs. 2010 Apr;15(4):S18-24. doi: 10.12968/bjcn.2010.15.Sup3.47365. PMID: 20559172.

Wixtrom R, Glicksman C, Kadin M, Lawrence M, Haws M, Ferenz S, Sung J, McGuire P. Heavy Metals in Breast Implant Capsules and Breast Tissue: Findings from the Systemic Symptoms in Women-Biospecimen Analysis Study: Part 2. Aesthet Surg J. 2022 Aug 24;42(9):1067-1076. doi: 10.1093/asj/sjac106. PMID: 35474526; PMCID: PMC9400612.

Yang S, Klietz ML, Harren AK, Wei Q, Hirsch T, Aitzetmüller MM. Understanding Breast Implant Illness: Etiology is the Key. Aesthet Surg J. 2022 Mar 15;42(4):370-377. doi: 10.1093/asj/sjab197. PMID: 33871569.

Yin L, He Z, Yi B, Xue L, Sun J. Simvastatin Suppresses Human Breast Cancer Cell Invasion by Decreasing the Expression of Pituitary Tumor-Transforming Gene 1. Front Pharmacol. 2020 Nov 4;11:574068. doi: 10.3389/fphar.2020.574068. PMID: 33250768; PMCID: PMC7672329.

Zhang JM, An J. Cytokines, inflammation, and pain. Int Anesthesiol Clin. 2007 Spring;45(2):27-37. doi: 10.1097/AIA.0b013e318034194e. PMID: 17426506; PMCID: PMC2785020.

Zikiryakhodzhaev AD, Alekseeva GS, Reshetov IV, Starkova MV, Saribekyan EK, Usov FN, Vlasova MY. Botulinum Toxin Type A as a Tool for Correcting Capsular Contracture after Reconstructive Breast Surgery. Plast Reconstr Surg Glob Open. 2021 Jan 25;9(1):e3372. doi: 10.1097/GOX.0000000000003372. PMID: 33552818; PMCID: PMC7861963.

Zingaretti N, De Biasio F, De Lorenzi F, Massarut S, Parodi PC. An efficient method for the correction of iatrogenic symmastia: A case series. Ann Med Surg (Lond). 2018 Mar 29;29:14-18. doi: 10.1016/j.amsu.2018.03.024. PMID: 29692891; PMCID: PMC5911666.

Made in the USA
Monee, IL
04 November 2026

67385846R10144